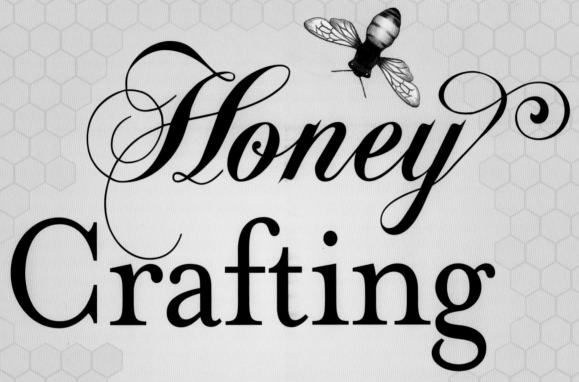

Honey Crafting

From DELICIOUS HONEY BUTTER *to* HEALING SALVES,
PROJECTS *for* YOUR HOME STRAIGHT *from the* HIVE

Leeann Coleman and Jayne Barnes

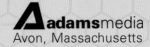
adamsmedia
Avon, Massachusetts

Published by
Adams Media, a division of F+W Media, Inc.
57 Littlefield Street, Avon, MA 02322. U.S.A.
www.adamsmedia.com

ISBN 10: 1-4405-5754-3
ISBN 13: 978-1-4405-5754-5
eISBN 10: 1-4405-5755-1
eISBN 13: 978-1-4405-5755-2

Printed in China.

10 9 8 7 6 5 4 3 2 1

Readers are urged to take all appropriate precautions before undertaking any how-to task. Always read and follow instructions and safety warnings for all tools and materials, and call in a professional if the task stretches your abilities too far. Although every effort has been made to provide the best possible information in this book, neither the publisher nor the author is responsible for accidents, injuries, or damage incurred as a result of tasks undertaken by readers. This book is not a substitute for professional services.

Always follow safety and commonsense cooking protocol while using kitchen utensils, operating ovens and stoves, and handling uncooked food. If children are assisting in the preparation of any recipe, they should always be supervised by an adult.

Many of the designations used by manufacturers and sellers to distinguish their product are claimed as trademarks. Where those designations appear in this book and F+W Media was aware of a trademark claim, the designations have been printed with initial capital letters.

Illustrations by Claudia Wolf.
Photographs by Stephanie Hannus except on pages 95, 117, 125, and 129 copyright © Stockfood; pages 4, 27, 86, 145, and 147 copyright © 123RF.com; pages 25, 89, 101, 104, 110, and 149 copyright © iStockphoto.

This book is available at quantity discounts for bulk purchases.
For information, please call 1-800-289-0963.

Contains material adapted and abridged from:

The Everything® Guide to Living Off the Grid, by Terri Reid, copyright © 2011 by F+W Media, Inc., ISBN 10: 1-4405-1275-2, ISBN 13: 978-14405-1275-9.

The Everything® Soapmaking Book, 2nd Edition, by Alicia Grosso, copyright © 2003, 2007 by F+W Media, Inc., ISBN 10: 1-59869-229-1, ISBN 13: 978-1-59869-229-7.

The Everything® Candlemaking Book, by M. J. Abadie, copyright © 2002 by F+W Media, Inc., ISBN 10: 1-58062-623-8, ISBN 13: 978-1-58062-623-1.

The Everything® Guide to Herbal Remedies, by Martha Schindler Connors with Larry Altshuler, MD, copyright © 2009 by F+W Media, Inc., ISBN 10: 1-59869-988-1, ISBN 13: 978-1-59869-988-3.

The Everything® Tex-Mex Cookbook, by Linda Larsen, copyright © 2006 by F+W Media, Inc., ISBN 10: 1-59337-580-8, ISBN 13: 978-1-59337-580-5.

The Everything® Cookies and Brownies Cookbook, by Marye Audet, copyright © 2009 by F+W Media, Inc., ISBN 10: 1-60550-125-5, ISBN 13: 978-1-60550-125-3.

The Everything® Cooking for Two Cookbook, by David Poran, copyright © 2005 by F+W Media, Inc., ISBN 10: 1-59337-370-8, ISBN 13: 978-1-59337-370-2.

The Everything® Mediterranean Cookbook, by Dawn Altomari-Rathjen, LPN, BPS, and Jennifer M. Bendelius, MS, RD, copyright © 2003 by F+W Media, Inc., ISBN 10: 1-58062-869-9, ISBN 13: 978-1-58062-869-3.

The Everything® Healthy Meals in Minutes Cookbook, by Patricia M. Butkus, copyright © 2005 by F+W Media, Inc., ISBN 10: 1-59337-302-3, ISBN 13: 978-1-59337-302-3.

The Everything® Classic Recipes Book, by Lynette Rohrer Shirk, copyright © 2006 by F+W Media, Inc., ISBN 10: 1-59337-690-1, ISBN 13: 978-1-59337-690-1.

The Everything® Italian Cookbook, by Dawn Altomari-Rathjen, BPS, copyright © 2005 by F+W Media, Inc., ISBN 10: 1-59337-420-8, ISBN 13: 978-1-59337-420-4.

The Everything® Ice Cream, Gelato, and Frozen Desserts Cookbook, by Susan Whetzel, copyright © 2012 by F+W Media, Inc., ISBN 10: 1-4405-2497-1, ISBN 13: 978-1-4405-2497-4.

The Everything® Indian Cookbook, by Monica Bhide, copyright © 2004 by F+W Media, Inc., ISBN 10: 1-59337-042-3, ISBN 13: 978-1-59337-042-8.

The Everything® Healthy Cooking for Parties Book, by Linda Larsen, copyright © 2008 by F+W Media, Inc., ISBN 10: 1-59869-925-3, ISBN 13: 978-1-59869-925-8.

The Everything® Cookbook, by Faith Jaycox, Sarah Jaycox, and Karen Lawson, copyright © 2000 by F+W Media, Inc., ISBN 10: 1-58062-400-6, ISBN 13: 978-1-58062-400-8.

For the **FLOWERS**, the **BEES**, the **HONEY**, and the **WAX**.

For the **CRAFTERS**, the **KEEPERS**, the **CHEFS**, and the **DREAMERS**.

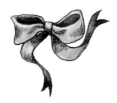

Contents

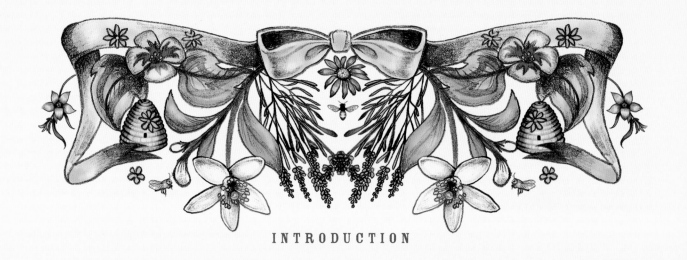

All of the Sweetness, None of the Sting

What is more glorious than honey? And what is more miraculous than the bees that make it?

On a warm day, the bees fly in and out of their hive. They flit from flower to flower, making our crops grow tall and our flowerbeds blossom lushly. Their affable buzzing is a genial and comforting background noise, the hum of a job done well.

Inside the hive, the bees are producing two of our dearest resources: honey and beeswax.

Honey is an ancient treasure, one that has been coveted and fought over since the days of cave people. Beeswax is as treasured and valuable to us as silk from a silkworm—a building block for our decorations and adornments. For as long as we have walked the earth, humankind has sought out the hive to reap the versatile wax and delectable syrup within.

In modern times, we are incredibly fortunate. These days, honey can be as near to us as our pantries, and busy hives can sit as close as our backyards. From the sprawling fields of the Midwest to the rooftops of New York City, enthusiastic beekeepers are discovering the delight of caring for their own busy colonies. With this providential surge of local hives comes a wealth of honey and beeswax to enjoy.

Honey Crafting will show you how to truly relish the fruits of the hive. In this book you'll find beeswax lanterns and candles that will paint the night with a honeyed, comforting glow. You'll find ornaments that could grace a wall or tree with a unique, natural embellishment, more striking and understated than glitter or gold.

You'll learn how to access the extraordinary health and beauty benefits of the hive as you craft honey soaps, moisturizing lip balms, and exfoliating facial scrubs. In *Honey Crafting* you'll find the key to making thick nourishing salves and syrups that will help to heal everything from sunburn to the common cold.

More nutritious than sugar, more versatile than maple syrup, honey is a staple of the kitchen. The recipes you'll find in this book take honey to new heights. Included are dramatic infusions with chili and ginger, savory glazes for tender meats and caramelized vegetables, and sweet honey pastries that will have you licking your fingertips.

All these crafts will bring you back to the hive. When you see the glow of a beeswax candle, touch a lip balm to your mouth, or taste the thick elixir of honey on your tongue, you'll be instantly transported. Even in the dead of winter, you'll be able to feel the sun warming your skin, hear the industrious buzz of winged creatures at work, and see the outline of a honeybee against a brilliant blue sky as it flies from the hive to your doorstep.

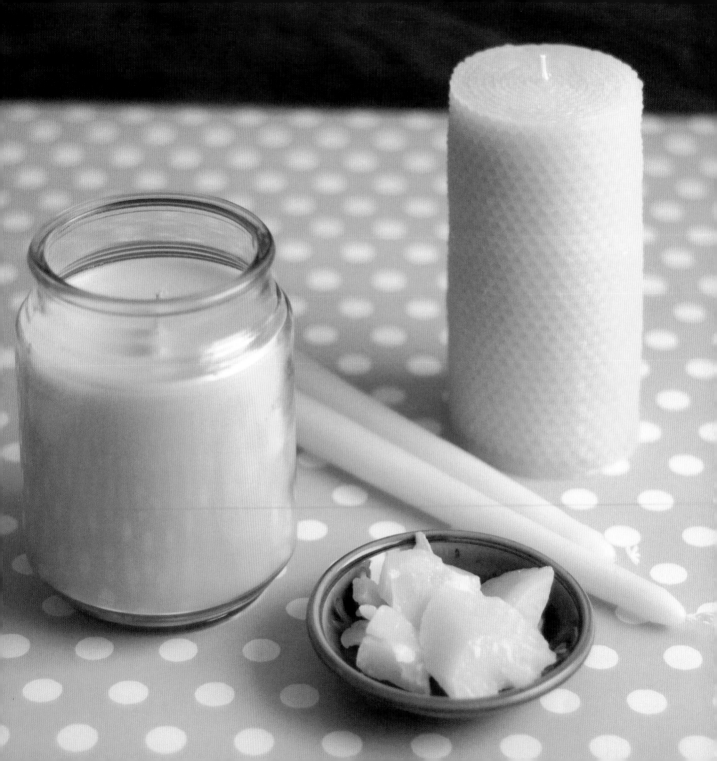

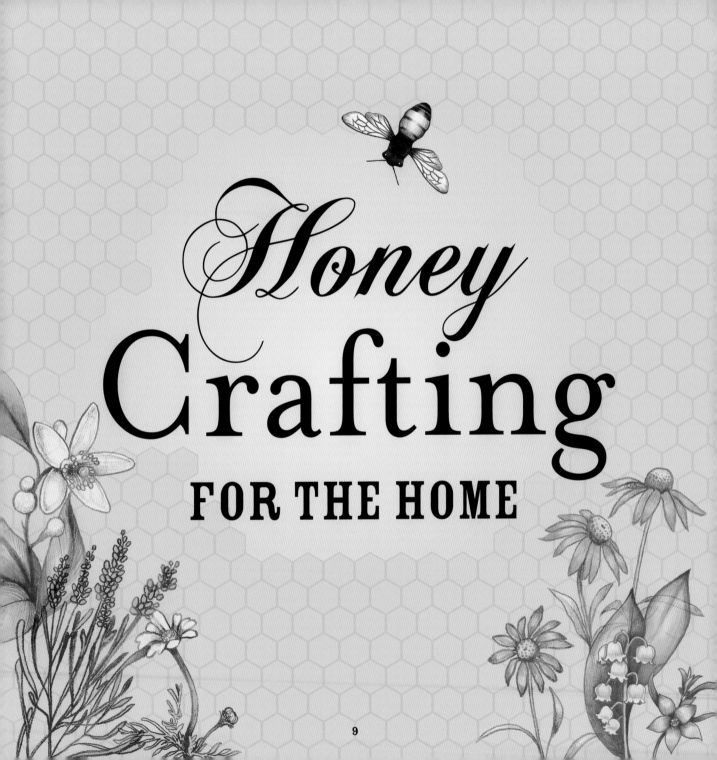

Honey
Crafting
FOR THE HOME

Introduction

Beeswax is so elegant, so lovely and useful, that it's hard to believe that it wasn't invented for us to enjoy.

In fact, beeswax is a product of the industrious worker bees, who use it to build honeycombs. That hexagonal pattern is actually a nursery for the hive's young and a pantry for the bees' pollen and honey. Wax is the building block of the hive.

And we, too, can use it to build. Of all the waxes that you can use to craft, pure beeswax is the most prized, and for good reason. Beeswax is a miracle of a medium for crafters. It's pliable when warm and sturdy when cooled. The soft yellow color of the beeswax seems to glow from within. It immediately draws the eye. Even a small beeswax candle or ornament can become the focal point of a living room or bedroom.

When formed into a candle and lit, the wax emits a rich, sweet fragrance that speaks to its enduring popularity. Each batch of beeswax has its own unique scent, a prized combination of the flowers and plants that fed its parent hive. Underneath the sweetness, look for notes of wildflowers, clover, avocados, or herbs in your beeswax.

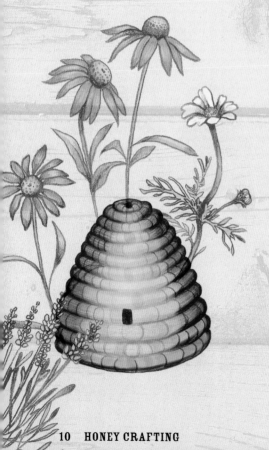

Beeswax burns with a pure, golden glow that nothing else can match, as the honeyed smell permeates the house and the occupants' hair and garments.

In Honey Crafting for the Home, you will find instructions on how to make your own beeswax masterpieces that will fill your home with beauty and light. Here you'll learn to craft candles of all shapes, sizes, and levels of difficulty. You'll find beeswax lanterns that could illuminate a living room with a joyous glow, and ornaments that could grace a tree or add class to the rear window of a car.

Honey Crafting for the Home will give you endless reasons to spend a night in with your new décor, and endless gifts for friends and family to celebrate.

Supplies and Safety

The crafts you'll learn to make in this section will lend splendor and substance wherever you display them. Beeswax is the most valuable and sophisticated crafting material on the market. That's because bees put so much effort into its production—they fly 150,000 miles and make 10 pounds of honey just to create a single pound of beeswax.

So it's important to act wisely when using it, lest you waste or even hurt yourself with the material that so many bees worked so hard to make. By having the correct supplies and following some basic safety protocols, you'll create beautiful and useful pieces of art that will honor the hives the wax came from.

SAFETY TIPS FOR BEESWAX

Before you begin to work with wax, it must be heated to its particular melting point. Take care not to overheat your wax. The "burning point" of wax is that temperature at which the properties of the particular wax have been stretched beyond the safety mark. Never leave melting wax on the heat source unattended—it is as volatile as cooking oil and can catch fire if overheated. Always keep a large pot lid handy to smother a fire, should one start. Also keep damp cloths handy for the same purpose.

Waxes are highly flammable—that's why candles burn! The temperature at which they will combust is the "flash point." This is approximately 440°F, depending on the type of wax you use. Never heat wax to the flash point. Watch your thermometer carefully.

If your wax does catch fire, stay calm and do the following:

- Turn off heat immediately. Do not move the pan.
- Smother flames with a metal lid or damp towel.
- Never use water to put out a wax fire.

Remember that the wax you are pouring is hot, and that it can burn you if spilled on your skin. Don't pour when you are feeling jittery or are distracted. Teach yourself to pour in a smooth steady stream by practicing first with water, using the vessel in which you plan to melt the wax.

It is also smart to have an ABC-type fire extinguisher on hand, as well as baking soda (dumped into a fire it will smother the flames immediately).

CLEANUP TIPS FOR BEESWAX

Don't ever pour liquid wax down your drain. It will solidify and cause severe blockage—not to mention a huge plumbing bill. Also, don't pour your hot double boiler water down your drain. It may have wax in it unbeknownst to you. Dispose of the water outside. Or, let it cool until the wax hardens and then remove the wax before pouring the water down the drain.

BEESWAX CRAFTING EQUIPMENT

Making the crafts in this section requires some basic equipment, most of which are neither expensive nor complicated. If you choose to use any of your cooking implements and/or pots for making candles, lanterns, or ornaments at home, dedicate any and all of that equipment to that end only. Not only will you avoid confusion, but you will also keep your food safe from contamination from wax, additives, dyes, and the like.

Thermometer

Your thermometer is vital. You can buy a special wax thermometer or use a candy or other cooking thermometer that covers a scale from 0°–300°F. It should have a clip so that you can immerse it deeply enough into your pot of melting wax to get an accurate reading.

Make sure your thermometer is accurate. You must always know the precise degree to which your wax has been heated. Check your thermometer regularly and discontinue use if it is no longer accurate.

Double Boilers

A system for melting wax is the primary consideration for many beeswax projects. For the novice crafter, the best melting method is the double boiler. Double boilers are extremely easy to improvise. You only need an outer pot to hold water and an inner pot in which to melt the wax. The outer pot must be large enough to hold an amount of water sufficient to rise two-thirds of the way up the inner pot. For the poured candles in this book, you can use a shallow round pot, big enough to melt as much wax as you will need. You can put one saucepan over another, or rest a fireproof bowl on a saucepan, but your wax may melt unevenly. Ideally, the inner pot will have a handle (a metal pitcher is excellent). A large can, such as the kind fruit juice is sold in, will work if you are willing to ladle out the wax. You can pour from such a can if you use mitts to protect your hands from the heat and are very careful.

If you improvise your double boiler, you will need a support for the inner pot, such as a metal trivet (the kind used on the dinner table to protect it from a hot dish). A support can be improvised as well, for instance by using three short cans (tuna fish or cat food cans will do). Cut out both ends and wire them together to make a three-pointed support. Or, cut out one end only and fill them with water so they don't float.

Remember to never put your wax-melting container directly on the heat source. And keep a careful watch on the water level in your outer pot. Don't let it boil dry. Add water frequently while melting wax.

You can also buy ready-made double boilers of many sizes. Cast aluminum and stainless steel double boilers for cooking are readily available wherever cookware is sold. As you'll see, most of these projects work best with stainless steel equipment, which best preserves the depth of color in beeswax.

Whichever kind of double boiler you use, you will need to replenish the water in the bottom pot frequently in order to keep your boiling water at the correct level. Your working surface must be level and have ready access to a water supply. You also need a heat source that is not an open flame. Your electric stove will work fine; a steady hot plate will suffice as well. Clean your melting vessel with paper towels after each use.

MISCELLANEOUS EQUIPMENT

As you honey craft for the home you'll find you need many supplies. These ancillary but necessary items are listed more or less in the order of importance, though all will eventually prove useful as you continue to expand your efforts. This list is not necessarily all-inclusive—you may think of other tools or implements that will be useful.

- **CAKE PANS AND COOKIE SHEETS.** Cake pans and cookie sheets are multipurpose. You can line them with nonstick pan spray or vegetable oil and pour unused melted wax in them to cool. They are also useful as pads for containers of hot wax.
- **SCALE.** A scale is an important piece of equipment as well, one you can't do without. Chances are you already have a kitchen scale that will do. It should have a range of 0–10 pounds, calibrated in ounces. You can use a gram scale. If you do, however, you will need to convert between grams and ounces and pounds. A scale is necessary for weighing not only wax but also additives such as stearic acid.
- **PYREX MEASURING CUPS.** These come in 1-cup, 2-cup, 4-cup, and 6-cup sizes, and are heat resistant. You can use the cups to determine the volume of wax by displacement. Put a block or chunks of wax in one cup; then put water in the second cup and note the amount it takes to fully submerge the wax in the first cup. Subtract the volume of water added from the level of water needed to cover the wax. The result is the volume of wax you have just measured. Because Pyrex measuring cups can be heated, you can also use such a measuring cup (or any heatproof calibrated vessel, such as a flask used in chemistry) as a wax-melting insert when melting small amounts of wax in an improvised double boiler.
- **OVEN MITTS AND POT HOLDERS.** Oven mitts or pot holders are essential for protecting your hands when you handle a pot of hot wax.
- **METAL RULER OR STRAIGHTEDGE.** An artist's T-square is good, as are the heavy metal rulers artists use. It's even a good idea to have both—for cutting and for calibrating lengths of vessels, candles, and wicks. These tools are available at art supply shops, which often also sell craft materials. You can use the straightedge to cut sheet wax for the rolled candles you'll learn about later in this chapter.
- **CUTTING SURFACE.** A cutting surface can be a laminated kitchen counter that can't be cut-marked, or a wooden or plastic cutting board such as those used for chopping food. You can even use a piece of heavy cardboard.
- **CUTTING TOOLS.** X-ACTO knives work well as cutting tools. The blades are extremely sharp and run cleanly along a straightedge. Use your cutting tool for cutting sheets of wax for rolled and stacked candles, and for trimming the seams of finished molded candles. Scissors are also useful, especially for cutting wicks.
- **STIRRERS.** Practically any old thing will do for stirring the melted wax, but old long-handled wooden spoons are ideal. If you don't have any, chances are you can pick up some cheaply at a garage or yard sale, or at a flea market. Another handy stirrer can

be had for free at your paint store. Paint stirrers are flat paddles given away with the purchase of paint, and paint store salespeople are usually happy to give you a few extra because the stirrers are imprinted with advertising for the brand of paint and/or the store. So when you have an occasion to buy paint, ask for extra stirrers and stash them away.

- **LADLE.** You might also need a ladle—choose one that's impervious to heat, with a deep bowl and a comfortably angled handle to avoid spilling.
- **GREASEPROOF PAPER AND PAPER TOWELS.** This includes waxed paper, parchment paper, brown craft paper (or brown paper bags flattened out), and foil. Keep a good supply on hand to cover work surfaces. And don't forget about paper towels—they are essential for cleanups, to use as oil wipes, to mop up water spills, and many other chores.
- **DOWELS.** When making a container candle, you'll need a straight rod of some kind to tie the wick to while you pour wax around it. Your dowel can be a chopstick or a piece of cardboard, anything that will support the weight of the wick.
- **WICK SUSTAINERS.** These little metal disks are used to anchor the wick in container candles, votives, and tealights. Wick sustainers are available wherever candle-making supplies are sold. To use, push the wick through a small hole in the sustainer and pinch the metal together so that it sits flat on the container base.
- **PAINT SCRAPER.** A paint scraper is excellent for easily scraping spilled wax off a hard surface, such as a counter. You might also use a putty knife.
- **WEIGHTS.** Small weights with a center hole are required to weigh down wicks that are being dipped. Washers, curtain weights, and nuts will all do.

Container Beeswax Candle

- 1 pound beeswax (amount will vary according to the size of your container)
- Double boiler designated for wax melting (preferably stainless steel)
- Wax or candy thermometer
- Pint glass jar or similar size container
- Wicking: Varies by size and type of container (see sidebar)
- Wick holder tab
- Glue

The container candle is the most versatile type of candle, with a long, storied history. If you look around your home, you're sure to find many glass jars with interesting shapes or attractive designs that you can utilize to make container candles. As your container candle burns and melts, the flame will flicker through the glass, illuminating your walls in delicate firelight.

Glass is the best material for containers. Ceramic or metal will also work, but those materials are opaque so you can't enjoy the glow as the candle burns down. Never use wood, milk cartons, or any other flammable materials for containers. Glass makes the loveliest kind of container, but be sure it is heavy enough not to crack under the burning candle's heat.

Container depth is important. Generally speaking, because the wick needs adequate oxygen to burn the candle properly, it's a good idea to select containers no more than 5 or 6 inches tall. Shorter ones—even very small ones—are ideal as they burn well and can be made in quantity and set around different areas of your rooms to give a candlelit feeling to the entire space. For example, baby food jars or other votive candle–size containers can be utilized this way. Try to pick containers that are either the same diameter at the top and at the bottom, or are wide-mouthed at the top. If your container does narrow at the neck, make sure your candle ends before that point.

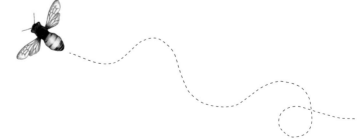

DIRECTIONS

1. Melt your beeswax using a double boiler—a small saucepan containing the beeswax, sitting inside a larger pan of water. Melting beeswax over direct heat is very dangerous, as hot beeswax is flammable and can ignite. Use a thermometer to monitor the temperature of your wax. Stainless steel pans are recommended because copper, brass, and iron can change the color of the wax, making it look dull.

2. Cut the length of your wick to extend beyond the top of your container.

3. When the beeswax has reached 150–160°F, prime your wick by dipping it in the beeswax until air bubbles stop releasing from the wick. Priming will allow the wick to stand straighter when placed in the container and aid in the initial lighting of the candle. Allow to dry.

4. Thread the wick through a wick holder tab.

5. Secure your wick tab to the bottom of your container using a dot of glue. Allow glue to dry.

6. If your vessel is a clear glass jar, it is recommended that you heat the jar by placing it in a 150°F oven prior to pouring. This will prevent the wax from pulling away from the side of the jar as it cools and shrinks, improving the overall appearance of the candle as seen through the outside of the jar.

7. Pour your candle when the wax has reached 150°F, using a slow, steady pour. Do not pour to the very top.

CANDLE DIAMETER AND WICK

- Less than 1 inch—4/0 wicking
- 1–3 inches—2/0 square braided wick
- Greater than 3 inches—1/0 square braided wick or 60 ply wicking

8. As the wax cools the wax surface will start to solidify. Pull the wick to the center to set it in place.

9. You will notice a sinkhole caused by shrinkage as the wax cools. Pour a second round of beeswax at a temperature of 155°F, just above the level of the original pour. This will cover the shrinkage and create a more even appearance at the top of the candle.

10. Allow the candle to cool and trim the wick to ¼ inch.

11. To dress up a plain container, consider tying colorful ribbons around the middle of the container, or drawing designs on the sides.

CANDLE IN AN ACORN

Natural materials and vintage containers can be used for container candles as well. Ideas include: a teacup, spice tins, orange peel, hollowed-out pumpkin or gourd shell, acorn caps (for floating in water), or sea shells. Be certain to follow the wicking guidelines from your wick supplier to ensure the proper size wick for the diameter of your candle.

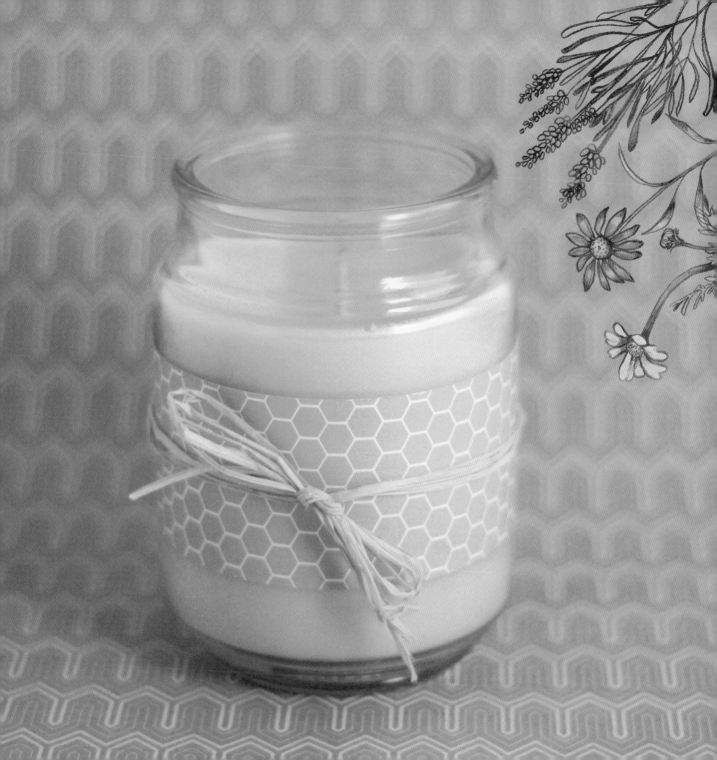

Beeswax Lantern

Usually we think of a burning beeswax candle as a fleeting delight, to be enjoyed and marveled at until it has burned down to a nub. But there are ways to craft with beeswax so that you can enjoy its presence forever.

This lantern is a particularly pleasant craft because it can be appreciated over and over again. Of course, you won't get the wonderful scent of beeswax when the lantern is lit—but you will have a warm glow that will cast intricate shadows against the walls.

Decorate the lantern with fall leaves for the perfect focal piece at the Thanksgiving table. Or cover it in seasonal flowers as a moving tribute to the pollen from which the beeswax came.

ITEMS NEEDED

- Balloon(s)
- Water faucet
- Double boiler designated for wax melting (preferably stainless steel)
- 1–2 pounds beeswax, depending on the size of the lantern
- Wax or candy thermometer
- Optional: Pressed leaves, flowers, or tissue paper for decorating the side of the lantern
- Aluminum foil
- Flat pan

DIRECTIONS

1. Begin by filling a balloon with water—this will serve as a form for your lantern. The size of your balloon will determine the size of your lantern. To ensure your balloon has a nice round shape, you may wish to blow up the balloon before filling it with water, to stretch out the sides and encourage the balloon to fill evenly.

2. Melt your beeswax using a double boiler—a small saucepan containing the beeswax, sitting inside a larger pan of water. Melting beeswax over direct heat is very dangerous, as hot beeswax is flammable and can ignite. Use a thermometer to monitor the temperature of your wax. Stainless steel pans are recommended because copper, brass, and iron can change the color of the wax, making it look dull.

3. When the wax has reached 150–160°F you are ready to begin dipping. Slowly dip your balloon with a slow and steady hand, immersing it for just a second. Remove it from the wax and allow it to dry, about 20 seconds. To speed up the process, you can alternate dipping back and forth between a bowl of cold water and the hot beeswax.

4. Continue to dip the lantern in wax a total of approximately 15–20 times, until desired thickness is reached.

5. If you would like to add decorations to the lantern, you can add pressed leaves, flowers, or tissue paper that has been cut into shapes. Dip the decoration in the beeswax, then carefully secure the edges of your decoration onto the side of your lantern with your fingers. Quickly dip the entire lantern one more time to secure the decorations with a thin coat of beeswax.

6. When the wax has cooled, turn your lantern upside down over a sink and snip the top of the balloon to remove it.

7. To finish the top and the bottom of the lantern, turn your stovetop on low and heat a flat pan. Cover the pan with aluminum foil, and touch the bottom of your luminary to the pan, slowly making circles to melt the wax on the bottom until it rests flat. Repeat the process for the top of the lantern to give it a nice smooth finish around the rim.

8. Your lantern is now finished and can be enjoyed indefinitely. Place a tealight in the bottom of the lantern to watch it glow. If your lantern is smaller than 4 inches wide, you will want to use a battery-powered tealight so the heat of the burning tealight does not melt the sides of your lantern.

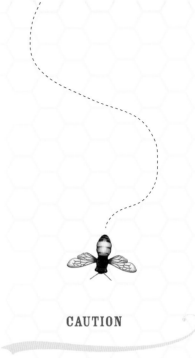

CAUTION

If your wax is too hot when you attempt to begin dipping, the balloon will pop and the wax will likely boil over the sides of your double boiler.

Hand-Dipped Beeswax Candle

ITEMS NEEDED

- 3 pounds of beeswax
- Double boiler designated for wax melting (preferably stainless steel)
- Wax or candy thermometer
- Wicking—2/0, approximately 30 inches for a pair of 10-inch candles
- 2 metal nuts or washers
- Dipping vat—a stainless steel vessel, at least 2 inches taller than the length of the candles you plan to dip

Imagine a special occasion candle—the kind that you put in an elegant silver holder for an anniversary dinner. These are the type of candles you burn while holding hands and staring deep into your partner's eyes. Long, tapered candles like these are made by hand dipping, one of the oldest methods of candle making.

Store-bought dipped candles may be made of a product called paraffin wax, an odorless petroleum byproduct that can be cheaply manufactured. Factories can add color and scent to paraffin candles, but they'll never match up to the beauty of a hand-dipped beeswax creation. By learning this hand-dipping method, you are ensuring that your special occasion candles will be truly exceptional.

DIRECTIONS

1. Melt the beeswax using a double boiler—a small saucepan containing the beeswax, sitting inside a larger pan of water. Melting beeswax over direct heat is very dangerous, as hot beeswax is flammable and can ignite. Use a thermometer to monitor the temperature of your wax. Stainless steel pans are recommended because copper, brass, and iron can change the color of the wax, making it look dull.

2. Cut your wicking to the length of candles desired, allowing extra room to tie washers or nuts to the end of each string. You will need approximately 30 inches for a pair of 10-inch candles.

3. Attach a nut or washer to each end of the wick; this serves as a weight, allowing the candle to stand straight while dipping.

4. When the wax has reached 150–160°F, prime the wick by holding it in the wax until the wick is thoroughly saturated and the wax is absorbed. Allow the primed wick to cool.

5. Keeping the temperature of the wax steady, dip the wicks again using a smooth movement, for about 3 seconds. Leave the dipped wicks to cool for approximately 3 minutes between dips.

6. Dip the candles approximately fifteen times, to the same point each time. This will form a nicely tapered tip. Keeping the wax heated at 155–160°F will give you a smoother finish, although it requires more dipping time.

7. After the final dip in beeswax, quickly dip the candle in water to give it a nice smooth finish.

8. Trim the bottom off the candle while it is still warm. The nuts or washers can be reused if you heat them in your melting pot to remove the hardened wax.

9. Allow the candle to cool for at least 1 hour before burning.

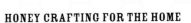

Molded Beeswax Ornaments

Beeswax ornaments can be made from a variety of flexible materials such as candy molds, cupcake tins, or molds made specifically for this purpose. These ornaments have a natural earthy appearance and look gorgeous swinging from an evergreen tree or hanging against a natural wood wall.

DIRECTIONS

1. Melt your wax using a double boiler—a small saucepan containing the beeswax, sitting inside a larger pan of water. Melting beeswax over direct heat is very dangerous, as hot beeswax is flammable and can ignite. Use a thermometer to monitor the temperature of your wax. Stainless steel pans are recommended because copper, brass, and iron can change the color of the wax, making it look dull.

2. When the wax reaches 160°F you may pour it into the molds. Pouring the wax at a temperature hotter than 160°F can ruin the molds, so be certain to monitor the temperature with the thermometer.

3. Cut your string to the appropriate length for hanging the ornament.

4. As the wax is starting to cool and you notice it firming at the edges, insert the two open ends of the string into the wax, holding it in place as the wax hardens. Be careful not to let the string fall toward the front of the mold where it will show through the front of the ornament.

5. After 3 hours your wax should be cool enough to remove from the mold. To make it easier to remove from the mold, place the mold in the freezer for several minutes after the wax has fully cooled, which causes the beeswax to shrink so it can be released more easily.

Over time, beeswax will develop a "bloom," which is a whitish coating over the outside of the wax. This is completely natural and harmless. Simply warm the wax with a hair dryer, or rub with a dry cloth to restore the original luster.

Rolled Tapered Beeswax Candle

ITEMS NEEDED

- Beeswax foundation or candle-rolling sheets
- Cutting board
- Ruler or measuring tape
- Knife for cutting the beeswax sheets
- 2/0 wicking (for candles 1–3 inches in diameter)
- Hair dryer

If the idea of crafting with hot wax makes you anxious, here is a craft that will produce splendid candles while easing your mind. The beeswax does not need to be melted down prior to working. This is also a wonderful way to bring children into the world of honey crafting. Imagine how proud young boys or girls would be to display their very own candles.

Sheets of beeswax were originally invented by beekeepers. These were, and still are, used to line the beehives. This wax liner gives the bees a firm foundation on which to build the honeycomb. Thus, the beekeepers call beeswax sheets "brood foundation." Beeswax candles can be made from foundation sheets.

Most wax sheets for rolled candles are formed in a honeycomb pattern. This type of sheet is embossed with a hexagonal indentation—it looks like the wax from a honeycomb. The most common size is 8″ × 16¾″, but you can cut the sheets to suit your specific purpose. The honeycomb-patterned sheets are rolled out under an embossing wheel. You can purchase these in the natural beeswax colors (pale honey to dark brown), or in various colors that they have been dyed after the wax was bleached.

Another type of wax for making rolled candles is smooth and flat. This is useful when you don't want a textured candle. The pure-white smooth sheets make an elegant-looking candle to use in a stylish setting.

DIRECTIONS

1. Lay the beeswax sheet on a cutting board and measure the halfway point on the long side (about 8½ inches). Cut vertically to separate the wax sheet into two pieces.

2. Cut your length of 2/0 wick to 9 inches and lay it against the 8-inch side of your beeswax sheet.

3. Using your fingers, pinch the edges of the beeswax around the wick, just enough to hold it firm and give you a nice edge to begin rolling.

4. Using a hair dryer on low heat, carefully blow back and forth across the beeswax sheet, holding the hair dryer about 2 inches from the wax. Depending on the strength of the hair dryer this will take approximately 30 seconds to 1 minute. You want the wax to begin to glisten, but not melt.

5. When the wax sheet is warm, you will begin rolling the candle, pushing away from you and using your rolled wick as the center. Use light, even pressure to maintain a nice rolled edge, being careful not to press the wax too firmly as it is warm.

6. When the candle is completely rolled it will fit perfectly in a standard tapered candlestick holder. Roll the second candle sheet in the same way, and you have a lovely pair of rolled beeswax tapered candles.

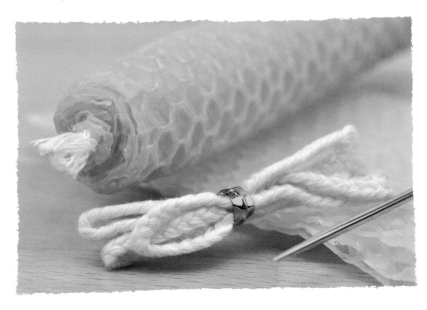

Square-Shaped Rolled Candle

ITEMS NEEDED

- 2/0 wicking (for candles 1–3 inches in diameter)
- Beeswax foundation or candle-rolling sheets
- Cutting board
- Knife for cutting the beeswax sheets
- Hair dryer
- Metal ruler
- Cookie sheet lined with paper
- 2 ounces melted beeswax

Once you have mastered the rolled tapered candle, you can experiment with different rolled shapes, creating an array of styles that would look magnificent lined up across a pastel shelf or down a mahogany table.

Using seven sheets of beeswax (9" × 12" each) and a primed wick 10 inches long, plus 2 ounces of melted beeswax, you can make a square candle from the textured sheets of beeswax. These are quite easy to make, with little mess as you only need to melt a small amount of wax.

DIRECTIONS

1. Lay the wick across one beeswax sheet as described previously in the instructions for Rolled Tapered Beeswax Candle. Roll up the entire sheet around the wick.

2. Place another sheet of beeswax next to the edge of the end of the first sheet and again roll tightly. Keep the edges even as you roll so that they remain the same length.

3. Using your metal ruler, press the sheets against a third sheet of beeswax at a 90-degree angle, pressing the roll into a square shape as you turn it over each time.

4. Continue adding the remaining sheets, using the ruler at each turn to make the sides square. After you have the edges shaped, lightly score each remaining sheet against the ruler to help you fold (not roll) the wax around the inner core of squared wax sheets.

5. Press the end of the final sheet firmly into place as you bend it around the candle. This step will ensure that the finished candle does not unroll as it burns.

6. Holding the finished candle upside down over a cookie sheet lined with paper to catch the drips, use a small spoon to pour some of the melted beeswax into the cracks between the layers of wax sheets. Smooth some melted wax evenly over the bottom to seal the candle together and give it a flat surface.

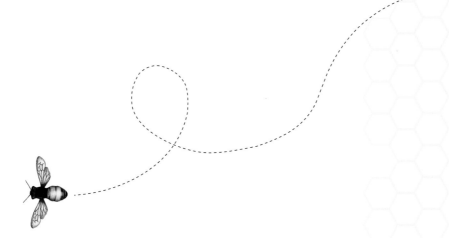

Cookie-Cutter Candle

ITEMS NEEDED

- Beeswax foundation or candle-rolling sheets—available in a variety of colors
- Cutting mat (this can be a cutting board or a piece of cardboard)
- Cookie cutters
- Hair dryer
- Square braided wick—2/0, for shapes under 3 inches wide

Most kitchens have a dozen or so cookie cutters that are used only once a year, if at all. With this craft, you'll be able to get use out of an old cutter and create a distinct and original candle that will last far longer than any cookie.

By using cookie cutters, you also open yourself up to an infinite wealth of choices. Once upon a time your shape options were limited to a star, a tree, or a gingerbread man. Now there are thousands of shapes to choose from. Try birthday candles in the shape of a child's favorite animal or bottle candles for a baby shower.

DIRECTIONS

1. Lay your beeswax sheet on the cutting mat. Using cookie cutters, cut out ten identical shapes.

2. Gently warm the beeswax shapes using a hair dryer. Press five of the shapes together so they adhere to each other. Using alternating colors will add interest to the appearance of the candle. Create two stacks of five shapes each.

3. Cut a length of 2/0 wick to extend 1 inch above the middle of your stacks. Line the wick up in the center of the cut-out stack and press the two stacks together to form your candle.

4. Trim the wick to extend ½ inch above the top of the shaped candle.

5. Adjust the base of your candle as needed to make it sturdy, or create a platform from excess layered beeswax sheets.

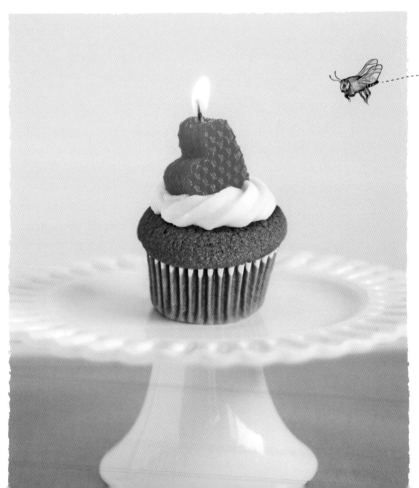

Making Your Own Wax Sheets

ITEMS NEEDED

- A piece of plywood the size of the wax sheet you want
- Beeswax
- A large, deep pot for melting the wax—a deep steamer of the type used for asparagus or corn will work, as will a deep stockpot
- Tongs or pliers

Although using purchased wax sheets is the easiest way to make rolled candles, if you are adventurous—and if you have some leftover wax from your container candle that you want to make use of—you can make your own wax sheets. Remember, a homemade wax sheet won't have the honeycomb pattern seen on the kind you can purchase.

DIRECTIONS

1. To prepare the plywood, soak it in water for an hour or more (to prevent it from absorbing the hot wax).

2. Dip the plywood into the melted wax, using tongs or pliers to hold it firmly. Allow the wax-covered plywood to cool for about a minute. Dip the wax-covered board into the wax again, and again allow it to cool. Repeat this process five or more times depending on the thickness of the wax sheet you want.

3. Scrape the wax at the edges of the board; then peel off the sheet.

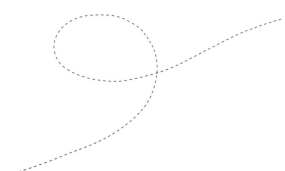

Homemade wax sheets lend themselves to various uses. Although purchased sheets come in lots of colors, you can tint your own wax sheets any color you like, or make multicolored layers for an interesting effect.

What's nice about homemade sheet wax is that you don't have to warm it up before using it. It will be warm when you remove it from the board. While it is still warm, you can form it into different shapes as you roll it.

Should the wax cool too much, just drop it into hot water (100–110°F) for a minute or two to soften it again. Keep a pot of warm water at hand for this purpose.

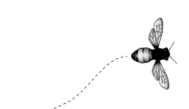

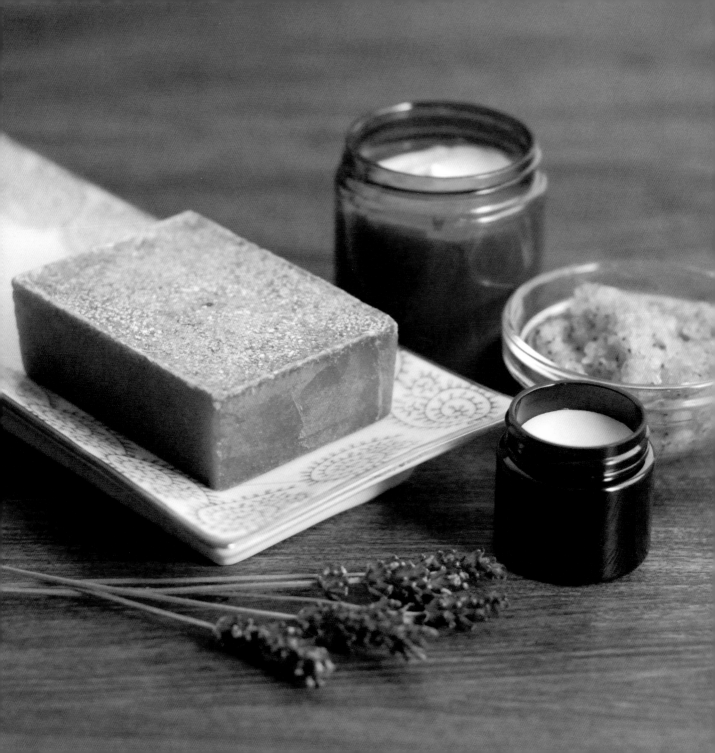

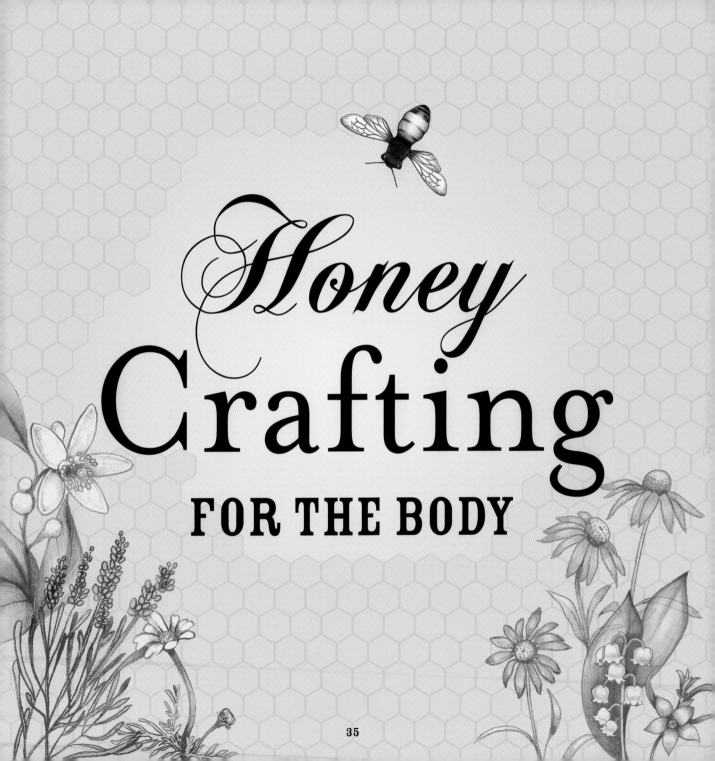

Honey
Crafting
FOR THE BODY

Introduction

In the last chapter, you found crafts that let you explore the role beeswax can play in your home's décor—delivering ambience and light to any room. If that were all the hive had given us, that would be enough. But beeswax and honey do more than delight our eyes and capture our imaginations. They also keep us healthy, strong, and vibrant.

After a day among the hives, beekeepers came home tired and worn. But they had at their fingertips the very materials that would restore bloom to their cheeks, shine to their skin, and moisture to their lips. Honey and beeswax are important elements in the most sumptuous bath and beauty supplies.

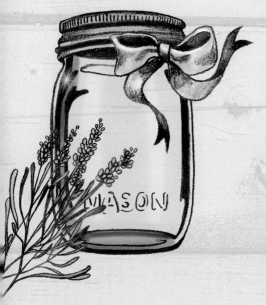

In Honey Crafting for the Body, you will learn how to make fragrant, gentle soaps to enjoy in a luxurious bath as well as hard-working, thorough soaps that will clean away even tough dirt and dust. You'll learn how to use the emollient properties of the hive's harvest to create a variety of lip balm flavors and textures. You'll also find instructions for creams and scrubs that will keep your skin firm and glowing. And you'll learn how to harness the hive's healing properties to make salves and syrups that will strengthen your heart, clear your chest, and soothe your scrapes.

With the embarrassment of riches that the hive supplies, you'll be able to make yourself a cure for various ills, from a bad cough to dry skin. Make more than you'll use, and put together bee-inspired gift baskets for your dearest friends and family. You can probably think of any number of people who deserve a relaxing spa day. With your honey-crafted goodies, they can get their day of relief without even leaving their homes.

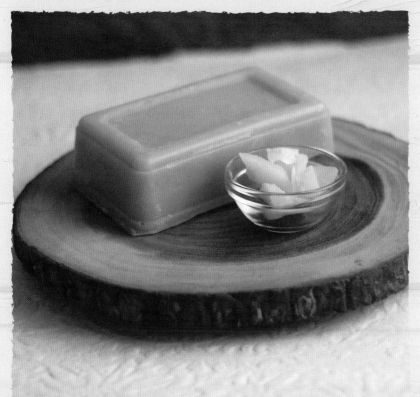

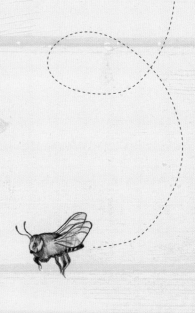

Supplies and Safety

In any new crafting endeavor, taking the time to obtain the proper equipment will make everything else go more smoothly. But this is especially important for some of the soap crafts covered in this chapter, because you'll be working with heat and caustic chemicals.

If you don't think you can safely keep and use soap-making materials in your environment, consider the melt-and-pour soaps and other projects in this chapter. But by following instructions and using safety gear, you should be able to make beautiful products out of honey and beeswax easily and safely.

SAFETY USING LYE

All soap is made with a caustic called lye. For the castile soaps in this book, you will use lye made of sodium hydroxide (chemical formula NaOH). Sodium hydroxide is readily available in 18-ounce plastic cans at grocery, hardware, and restaurant supply stores. Do not buy anything other than pure sodium hydroxide. The safest way to purchase lye is from soap-making suppliers.

Store lye in a safe, dry place—under the kitchen sink is not a good idea, especially if you have kids. Many home soapers have a "lye safe" just for lye storage. Lye safes can range from a box in the garage clearly marked "Lye! Do Not Touch!" to a metal cabinet with locking doors. Storing your lye safe on a high shelf isn't recommended—you could easily drop it, especially if you keep more than a few pounds at home.

In your lye safe, keep the plastic cans of lye in plastic bags. Take care how you dispose of empty containers. Neutralize the lye dust by rinsing the containers with a vinegar-and-water solution. If you have a hazardous material drop-off day in your community, take your empty lye cans to the collection point.

Combining lye with water creates an extremely violent, volatile chemical reaction. It is *essential* that you add the lye to the water rather than the water to the lye. The lye releases a great deal of energy in the form of heat immediately upon contact with water. If you pour cold water on top of lye, you could end up with a volcano-like eruption that would be extremely dangerous. When you add water to lye, the chemical reaction causes the solution to heat almost immediately to nearly boiling. If water is poured onto the lye, it forms a crust over the top of the lye, which seals in the reaction below. The reaction of the lye and water proceeds normally but in a confined space, causing a buildup of heat energy that eventually bursts open like a bomb, showering the area with dangerously caustic material. Never use aluminum or copper when working with lye, it will cause a reaction. Instead use Pyrex, which is safer.

Never add lye to a hot liquid. The reaction is so violent and rapid that you'll be dangerously close to or over the boiling point in no time. Even when you correctly add lye to water, do so with care. The solution will heat up very fast and will steam. Do not breathe the steam. Usually it is enough just to stand back and not breathe the steam, but if you are concerned about sensitivity to lye steam, look into purchasing a chemical respirator. If you are mixing lye on your stovetop, consider running the exhaust fan if you have one.

The lye-and-water solution will heat up to about 180°F. You need to let the solution cool before combining it with the prepared oils. Soap-making temperatures can range from room temperature (so long as the room is warm enough to keep the oils liquid) to as high as 150°F. If you are a beginner, you may wish to allow the solution's temperature to go a bit lower, perhaps to 120°F, before taking the next soap-making step.

You can take the steaming lye solution outside to let it cool. Just be sure it is in a safe place where no one can get to it and it won't get knocked over. It is also a good idea to cover the container so no leaves or other debris fall into it.

All this can be alarming, and potentially dangerous, but if you pay attention and use your head, you'll be perfectly safe. Lye soap is made at home all the time in complete safety. Your safety depends on the use of common sense. If you plan well, everything will go smoothly. The more soap you make, the more you will tailor your safety practices to your situation. Safety essentials are goggles, rubber gloves, and an apron.

SAFETY DURING CURING

Curing refers to the period after cutting, during which the soap becomes milder and harder—milder as saponification finishes and harder as water evaporates. You can extend the life of your soap through careful formulation and storage. Over time, expo-sure to heat and humidity can degrade the quality of your soaps. Soap that sits in water or is allowed to languish in the stream of the shower will melt away rapidly, so dry your soap between uses.

After cutting and while curing, soap needs to be kept at a relatively constant temperature and have air circulation. Depending on the amount of soap you make, you can dry your soap on a paper-covered cookie sheet or a small shelf. Or, create an entire curing and drying rack system. However you choose to cure it, be sure to turn it every few days during the first couple weeks so that it will cure evenly.

As mentioned earlier, lye is extremely caustic. When you first add the lye to the liquid, the resulting solution is also extremely caustic. After this lye solution is mixed with the soap-making oils, however, the soap begins to neutralize, and becomes safe to touch after it has cured. Always wear goggles and rubber gloves when handling lye, lye solutions, raw soap, and fresh soap. If you are in doubt about how neutralized your soap is, err on the side of wearing goggles and gloves even when they're not needed.

Testing for Neutrality

You can test for neutrality of soap in a number of ways. Using phenolphthalein or litmus papers is the most popular. Phenolphthalein is very reliable, inexpensive, and easy to use. You simply place a couple drops of the solution on the soap you are testing. If the solution turns pink, it is alkaline. If it stays clear, it is neutral.

You can purchase litmus kits online and at your garden center. Follow the directions on the kit. Often you'll be instructed to use a color comparison chart on the box. You can also purchase an electronic pH meter. Soap is "safe" when it registers between 7 and 10 on the pH scale.

Handling Caustic Messes

While your soap is curing, test it every so often for neutrality. If your soap is more than 2 weeks old and is still highly caustic, something went wrong and the soap should not be used. Find out from your city or county what the proper disposal method is for caustic materials.

Keep a caustic mess contained until you can dispose of it properly. Line a heavy cardboard box with two heavy plastic garbage bags, one inside the other. Fill the box with clay kitty litter deep enough to absorb the mess. Wearing goggles and gloves, pour or scrape the caustic mess into the bags. Add an equal measure of vinegar. If the mess is soupy, add more litter. Label the box and store it in a safe place until you can dispose of it.

SAFETY DURING CLEANUP

Be sure you don't rinse large blobs of gooey soap, either finished or unsaponified, down your drains. They will clog your drains.

Because the soap is caustic all the way through the process and for a few weeks after, always wear goggles and gloves while handling it.

Keep track of all the utensils and equipment that you've used with the lye. Rinse the lye-pouring pitcher with water and a splash of vinegar, set it in the kitchen sink, then fill it partway with water and more vinegar so you can place the other things in a neutralizing bath. Be sure not to hit it with a hard stream of water that will splatter. After you're finished with a lye-touched tool, put it in the pitcher. Keep adding the utensils as you finish, pouring vinegar on them as you go.

After you've scraped the last of the beautiful soap batter into the molds, wipe the inside of the pan and any other tools you've used. You can use paper towels, but you'll go through a lot of them. A better idea is to get old cloth towels out of the ragbag and tear them into paper towel–sized soap cleanup towels. To reuse, place the towels in a plastic bag for a day or two, then add them to the wash. The soap will have saponified enough for laundry use and will contribute to the cleansing.

STOCKING YOUR SOAP-MAKING SUPPLIES

If you research and shop carefully, you can outfit yourself for these projects for far less money than you might think.

EYE PROTECTION. Make sure that the eye protection you use is resistant to impact, caustics, and heat. If you wear glasses, get goggles that are large enough to wear over them. The danger to your eyes comes from the potential of lye particles, lye solution, raw soap, hot oils, and other liquids splashing you in the face. So long as you work mindfully, you will experience very few—if any—splashing events. However, you do not want to be caught unprotected if one should occur.

GLOVES. Regular rubber kitchen gloves provide appropriate protection for your hands and lower arms. Buy gloves with textured fingers so that you can keep a firm grip on your equipment. Some crafters prefer heavy-duty gloves. Just be sure you can use your fingers freely.

When you are finished with your soap-making project for the day, clean your gloves well with soap and water. If you clean and dry them regularly, they'll last quite some time. Turn them inside out to dry and store them only after they're completely dry.

To protect your arms above the gloves wear a long-sleeved shirt. An oversized button-up shirt with sleeves you can roll up is ideal.

VINEGAR. Vinegar has traditionally been used as a neutralizer for lye and raw soap spills, but you should not pour vinegar onto an alkaline spill on the skin. It would be a good idea to let your doctor know you are making soap, and ask about the best way to handle skin contact with caustics. If you come in contact with lye or raw soap batter, gently wipe the spill from your skin, then flush the area with water. Then you can douse the affected area with vinegar if desired. Flush again with water and finally wash with soap and water. Don't wait to finish stirring your batch before rinsing and neutralizing a smear of raw soap from your skin. Do it as soon as it gets on you.

SCALE. The best way to measure ingredients is by weight. Therefore, you will need a good scale. Digital postal scales, available at office supply stores, are the choice for many crafters. They usually run on 9-volt batteries, have the tare feature, weigh in ¼-ounce increments, and weigh up to a maximum of 10 pounds.

THERMOMETER. A good thermometer is key for the projects in this section, just as it is for the beeswax crafts in the previous chapter. You will need an instant-read thermometer. You may want to get two, in case you need to measure the temperatures of two containers at the same time.

POTS AND PANS. When buying your soap-making pots and pans, stainless steel is the way to go. You can find stainless steel pots and pans at extremely reasonable prices at restaurant supply, warehouse, discount, and thrift stores. You absolutely must not use nonstick, aluminum, cast iron, or tin. They will react badly—even violently and toxically—with the lye used in the soap-making process.

DOUBLE BOILER. The basic 2-quart, two-part stainless steel double boiler is perfect for the recipes in this book. You can improvise a double boiler using a saucepan and a stainless steel mixing bowl that rests securely but not tightly on the pan. (Always be sure when using any kind of double boiler not to let it boil dry.)

STAINLESS STEEL UTENSILS. Stainless steel stirring spoons, slotted spoons, potato mashers, and ladles are all very useful for soap crafting. You probably already have these in your kitchen, and it is safe to use them for your first few batches. So long as you clean them thoroughly, there is no danger in using them afterward because the metal does not readily absorb or react with the soap. If you find yourself making a great deal of soap, it may be easier to invest in stainless steel tools just for soaping.

Some stainless steel tools are held together with reactive metal screws, bolts, or brads. You probably won't be able to tell what type of metal the fasteners are, so choose utensils that are all one piece or have "all stainless construction" printed on the package. If you're in doubt, pass it by.

SILICONE UTENSILS. Silicone rubber scrapers, or what many people call "spatulas," are useful tools. Choose a one-piece model so you will never lose the scraper part in a batch of soap.

MEASURING EQUIPMENT. The small-batch, cold-process recipes in this book call for two 2-quart measuring cups or large bowls: one for mixing the lye solution and the other for mixing the oils and stirring the soap. You'll also need accurate measuring cups for the rest of the projects in this section, to measure honey for the syrups or oils for body creams. They are, of course, also always useful for

measuring water. It is tempting to use the attractive, thinner, heatproof glass, but just stick to the heavy-duty variety, as the thin glass will shatter.

Sets of stainless steel measuring cups and spoons can be used for all of the crafts in this section. It's best to steer clear of plastic measuring cups and spoons. Although they can be good for some things, they may be corroded by essential oils and fragrance oils or marred by heat.

SOAP MOLDS. From a clever and simple slab mold to incredibly detailed and delicate designs, the variety and quality of available soap molds will astound you. You can find both simple and elaborate molds online and from specialty soap suppliers.

You can buy single-bar molds in just about any design you can imagine. Some manufacturers make them in trays of three, four, or more. Others make single-cavity molds. Your best bet is to check out a large craft store or an online soap mold supplier. Molds that are made especially for soap making will have information regarding the method of soap making—cold-process, melt-and-pour, etc.—for which they are best suited. Always test a new mold for heat resistance before using it the first time. Pouring time is too late.

You might want to make your own molds. Shoeboxes lined with plastic bags, baby-wipe containers, inexpensive plastic storage containers, and other everyday receptacles have all been pressed into service as soap molds. You can even use tubes from paper towels or toilet paper rolls.

Empty plastic wrap and aluminum foil boxes can serve as small, lidded molds. If you're using something plastic for a mold, such as a baby-wipe container, be sure to test it for heat resistance. Because of the high temperatures involved in soap making, you need plastics that will not collapse when exposed to hot soap. The easiest way to check a mold for heat safety is to place it in the sink and fill it with boiling water. If it melts, it is obviously not going to be useful. If it warps and distorts, it is not a good choice either. If you decide to make a basic mold from a cardboard box lined with a plastic garbage bag, be sure the box will hold the soap batch. Measure an equivalent amount of water and pour it into the lined mold. If it doesn't fit, keep testing until you get just the size box you want.

PUMP CONTAINERS FOR LIQUID SOAP. Transparent, squeezable plastic bottles that are made of PET plastic are ideal for holding aromatic oils. Many kinds of plastic will not stand up to fragrance oils or essential oils. Look for the initials PET (which stand for polyethylene terephthalate) on the bottom of the bottles if you reuse bottles you already have or buy them at the drug store. If you order from an online soap-making supplier, read the product descriptions to be sure you get PET.

CUTTING TOOLS. The simplest soap cutter is a stainless steel table knife. Most soapers prefer nonserrated-edge knives because they make a clean cut. Dough scrapers borrowed from baking, and putty knives and drywall tape spreaders borrowed from home improvement work very well, too.

ADDING SCENT TO YOUR SOAP

When you pick up a bar of soap, the first thing you probably do is hold it to your nose and sniff. The packaging, color, and other visuals may attract you, but it's likely the scent that captures or repels you. Some people choose unscented products all or some of the time. Two of the easiest ways to scent your soap are to add essential oils or fragrance oils. When you create blends using both essential oils and fragrance oils, you need to be sure you use the proper measurements for each. Fragrance oils are usually added at about one-third the rate of essential oils. Not all fragrance oils are the same potency, so be sure you get the manufacturer's or distributor's rate of use for each oil you use.

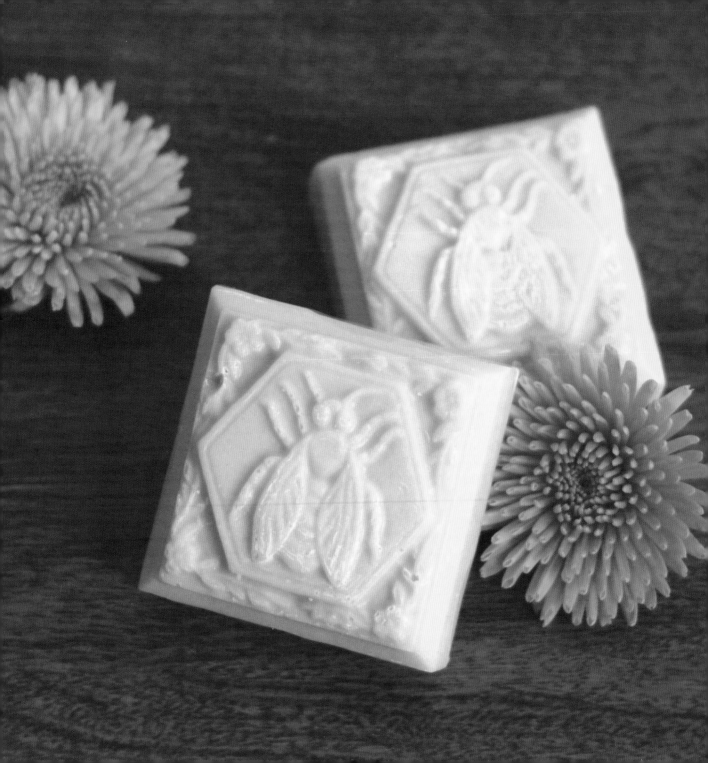

Castile Soap

Castile soap is the most basic and gentlest of all soaps, made from a simple recipe of saponified olive oil and beeswax. The soap has no lather, but provides excellent, gentle cleaning. The beeswax in this recipe makes the bars hard and long lasting. Doctors often recommend castile soap to their patients with allergy-prone or reactive skin types, as well as for babies. This is a basic recipe for a scentless soap.

IMPORTANT SAFETY NOTE

You should always take care when using lye. Lye, when added to water, creates a chemical reaction that produces heat. Be sure to protect countertops with a thick layer of newspaper. Lye is corrosive—never handle lye without eye and skin protection. Always use lye in a well-ventilated area.

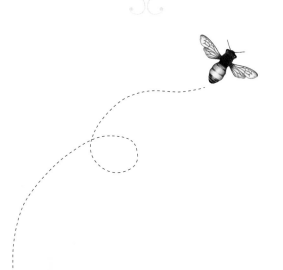

ITEMS NEEDED

- Rubber gloves
- Lab goggles or other eye protection
- Apron
- A small scale
- 1 cup distilled water, room temperature
- 2 large glass measuring cups (2-quart) or 2 heat-safe glass bowls
- 2¼ ounces (weight) lye
- Wax or candy thermometer
- 16 ounces (weight) pure olive oil
- 1 ounce (weight) beeswax
- Hand mixer or stick blender
- Rubber spatula
- Commercial soap molds, reusable-type plastic containers, or paper milk cartons lined with waxed paper to use as molds
- Plastic wrap
- Newspaper
- Thick towels to insulate your molds
- Knife

DIRECTIONS

1. Pour water into bowl.

2. Very carefully, pour the lye into the water while stirring. The lye will react with the water and produce heat. Set aside and allow the lye solution to cool to 150°F.

3. While the lye solution is cooling, prepare the oil solution. In the second large glass bowl, combine olive oil and beeswax. Microwave for 30 seconds and stir, repeating until beeswax is melted and the temperature of the liquid is 150°F.

4. Beat the oil mixture using hand mixer or immersion stick blender. While beating, carefully pour the lye mixture into the oil in a slow and steady stream. Mix for 5 minutes, scraping down the sides of the bowl frequently. The mixture will begin to thicken. In the soap world, this is called "trace." The term trace refers to the presence of traces of the soap mixture on the surface of the mass when some is taken up on your stirrer and dribbled back in. If the dribble makes no mark, your soap has not traced. When it leaves a little lump on the surface that sinks in quickly, it's beginning to trace. You must stir your soap to trace before pouring into the molds. If your soap hasn't traced, it will likely separate and remain unsaponified in layers of oils and lye solution.

5. When the mixture is the consistency of pudding, pour into prepared molds. Cover molds with plastic wrap, and then cover that with several thick towels; set aside. The lye will continue to react in the soap mixture for a few days—the goal is to cool the soap slowly.

6. After 3 days, uncover soap and unmold. Cut into slices if necessary. Allow the soaps to dry out and cure in an undisturbed place for 6 weeks before using them, turning the pieces over once or twice a week.

UNMOLDING TIPS

Soapmakers struggle with unmolding all the time. A simple way to ensure easy release is to line the bottom and sides of the mold. You could brush vegetable oil lightly on the inside of the mold. Then cut plastic sheeting, freezer paper, overhead projector transparency, or other similar materials to size and press onto the oiled surface. Smooth out bumps and creases in the liner to ensure smooth surfaces on your soap.

When the soap is ready to unmold, if all has gone as it should, all you'll have to do is turn the mold over and the beautiful soap will just fall out onto the table. If, after a few days, the soap won't release from the mold, put it in the freezer for half an hour and try again.

Chamomile Castile Soap

- 1 quart olive oil
- 2 cups dried chamomile flowers
- Crockpot
- 1 cup distilled water
- 2 large (2-quart) glass measuring cups or 2 heat-safe glass bowls
- Rubber gloves
- Lab goggles or other eye protection
- Apron
- A small scale
- 2¼ ounces (weight) lye
- Wax or candy thermometer
- 1 ounce (weight) beeswax
- Hand mixer or immersion stick blender
- Rubber spatula
- Molds
- Plastic wrap
- Newspaper
- Thick towels to insulate your molds
- Knife

Once you've mastered the basic beeswax castile soap, you can branch out and take advantage of the herbal benefits that soap can offer. Chamomile is particularly good for sensitive skin. It possesses anti-inflammatory properties that can provide relief from irritation. Chamomile also rejuvenates the skin, decreases puffy eyes and dark circles under the eyes, and significantly reduces wrinkles and brown spots on the face.

For a chic touch, give this soap an unusual look and a lovely texture by adding chamomile flowers to the soap before pouring the concoction into your molds.

DIRECTIONS FOR INFUSION

1. To make the infusion, place 1 quart olive oil and 2 cups dried chamomile flowers in crockpot.

2. On low setting with the lid cracked open to allow any moisture to escape, allow mixture to heat overnight.

3. The next day remove the infused oil and let it cool.

4. Strain out the solid flowers, but keep them on hand if you'd like to use them for texture and decoration in the soap.

DIRECTIONS FOR SOAP

1. Measure room-temperature water; pour into bowl.

2. Very carefully stir lye into water. The lye will react with the water and produce heat. Set aside and allow the lye solution to cool to 150°F.

(See the instructions for Castile Soap or the safety section for information on safely using lye.)

3. While the lye solution is cooling, weigh out the 16 ounces of infused oil and combine it with the beeswax in the second large glass bowl. Microwave for 30 seconds and stir, repeating until beeswax is melted and the temperature of the liquid is 150°F.

4. Beat the oil mixture using hand mixer or stick blender. While beating, carefully pour the lye mixture into the oil in a slow and steady stream. Mix for 5 minutes, scraping down the sides of the bowl frequently. The mixture will begin to thicken, or "trace."

5. Once the mixture is the consistency of pudding, you can stir in the strained chamomile flowers if you wish.

6. Pour into prepared molds. Cover molds with plastic wrap, and then cover that with several thick towels. Set aside. The lye will continue to react in the soap mixture for a few days—the goal is to cool the soap slowly.

7. After 3 days, uncover soap and unmold. Cut into slices if necessary. Allow the soaps to dry out and cure in an undisturbed place for 6 weeks before using, turning the pieces over once or twice a week.

GIFTING IDEA: SMALL BOXES

Small boxes can be decorated to hold one or more bars of soap. You can find little boxes in office supply, jewelry supply, and packaging supply stores. Small folded takeout boxes, such as those often used by Chinese restaurants, are cute containers for bars of soap. Place a couple prettily wrapped bars in the container and make a label for the container out of the same paper you used to wrap the soap.

Balsam and Basil Soap

ITEMS NEEDED

- 3½ pounds opaque white melt-and-pour soap
- 2 tablespoons beeswax
- 2 teaspoons cocoa butter
- Double boiler
- 2 teaspoons balsam fragrance oil or evergreen scent
- 2 teaspoons lime essential oil
- 10 drops of vitamin E oil
- ¼ cup dried basil leaves, crushed
- Molds
- Plastic wrap

This soap has a woodsy, outdoorsy smell that evokes cozy winter nights.

Melt-and-pour soap casting is a wonderfully accessible method of making soap at home. A simple meltable soap base, commonly called glycerin soap base, can be recreated in a dazzling array of forms. If you have small children and are worried about having lye in your household, this is a lovely way to make soap without using caustics.

DIRECTIONS

1. Melt soap, beeswax, and cocoa butter in the top half of a double boiler; remove from heat.

2. Add 2 teaspoons each of fragrance oil and essential oil and stir until blended.

3. Add vitamin E and stir until blended.

4. Stir in basil leaves. Pour soap into molds.

5. Allow soap to cool completely, unmold, and wrap in plastic.

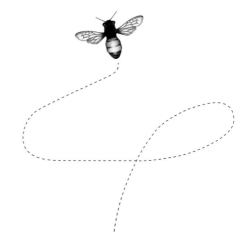

Gardener's Scrub Bar

After a day of digging and weeding, soil finds its way into every crevice of a gardener's skin. It sticks to cuticles and lodges in the webbing between fingers. Often, no matter how hard you scrub, the dirt still clings.

The citrus oil in this recipe, along with the texture provided by the poppy seeds and pumice, cuts through the soil and washes away even the most stubborn dirt. Meanwhile, the shea butter soothes your skin, which can get chapped and dry from pulling out tough weeds and hefting heavy flowerpots.

DIRECTIONS

1. Melt soap, stearic acid, and shea butter in the top of a double boiler.

2. Add poppy seeds, pumice, dried pulverized orange peel, ground chamomile, lemongrass oil, and orange oil.

3. Allow mixture to cool to 120°F and stir thoroughly before pouring into molds. This will allow the ingredients to remain suspended in the bar and not settle to the bottom.

4. Allow soaps to cool completely, then unmold.

5. Wrap each bar in plastic wrap.

ITEMS NEEDED

- 32 ounces melt-and-pour soap
- Double boiler
- ¾ ounce stearic acid
- 2 tablespoons shea butter
- 4 tablespoons poppy seeds
- 3 tablespoons pumice
- 1 tablespoon dried, pulverized orange peel
- 2 tablespoons ground chamomile flowers
- 2 tablespoons lemongrass essential oil
- 1 tablespoon orange essential oil
- Wax or candy thermometer
- Molds
- Plastic wrap

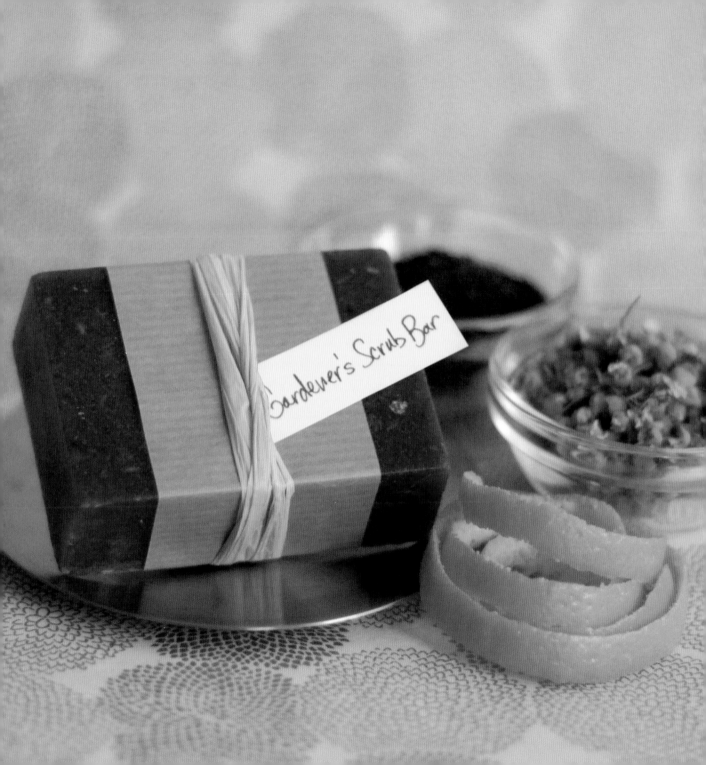

Gardener's Scrub Bar

GIFTING IDEA: THE CIGAR BAND WRAPPER

A simple "cigar band" wrapper is an elegant and easy way to wrap a bar of soap. The name of this style of wrap comes from the practice of placing a small ring of paper around a cigar to indicate the type and maker. You can create a band of paper on a larger scale to fit around your bar of soap.

To decide the size to cut the paper, measure around the bar with a tape measure or wrap a piece of paper or string around the bar and measure that. You will have an easier time fastening the ends of the paper if they overlap by about ½ inch. Sometimes you'll want to cover the bar end to end with a wide band, and other times you'll want a narrower band that doesn't conceal the soap.

The easiest way to fix the ends once you've wrapped the soap is with a small piece of clear tape. For a more finished look, use double-sided tape. Place the small piece of tape under one end of the band and press it down firmly to fix it to the other side. You can also use a glue stick to fasten the bands. Wrap the paper around the bar, and apply a small amount of glue to the inside of the overlapping edge. Press the glued side to the other side firmly.

Oatmeal and Honey Scrub Bar

ITEMS NEEDED

- 40 ounces white melt-and-pour soap
- Double boiler
- ½ cup rolled oats, chopped fine
- ½ teaspoon kaolin clay
- 2 tablespoons honey
- 2 teaspoons fragrance oil or essential oil
- Molds
- Plastic wrap

This bar features a surprising special effect that will delight whoever uses it. After you've poured the mixture into the mold, the clay and oatmeal will settle to the bottom. The end result is a dual-purpose bar with one smooth side for cleaning and one rougher side for exfoliating.

You may never have heard of kaolin clay, but you likely use it every day. It is a common substance in toothpaste, lightbulbs, and many cosmetics. You can purchase kaolin clay from most soap-making suppliers.

DIRECTIONS

1. Melt soap in the top of double boiler.

2. Once the soap is fully melted, add the oats, clay, honey, and oil.

3. Stir well and pour immediately into molds.

4. Allow soaps to cool completely, then unmold and wrap in plastic.

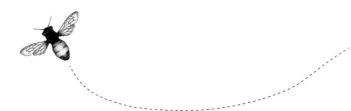

GIFTING IDEA: PLASTIC WRAP AND BAGS

You can use stretchy plastic cling film to wrap melt-and-pour soaps to protect them. Cut a square of wrap a few inches bigger than the bar. Place the bar in the middle, face down. Gather up the edges and gently pull the wrap tight over the surface of the bar. Twist tightly, cut close to the soap, and fix with a piece of tape or a sticker.

Remember that plastic wrap is not the best packaging for lye soaps, because they need to have air circulation to prevent spoilage. If you shrink-wrap them, use wrap that has tiny circulation holes and leave the ends unwrapped.

Stiff plastic bags commonly called "cellophane" bags are an excellent presentation material. You can tie the top with raffia, decorative yarn, or ribbon.

Liquid Soap

- Double boiler
- 2 cups grated, cured castile soap (from the Castile Soap instructions, found earlier in this section)
- 1 tablespoon olive oil
- 2 tablespoons vegetable glycerin
- 3 cups distilled water
- 1 teaspoon vodka
- 2 teaspoons of your favorite essential oil or fragrance oil
- 2 pump-style soap bottles, new or used

Liquid soap offers many advantages. You need not concern yourself with dropping a bar of your lovely handmade soap onto a dirty bathroom floor. Sometimes the gel of a liquid soap can ease into little niches of your body that would be difficult to clean with a large bar of hard soap. And you can control the amount of soap you're using, which is especially useful if you're teaching children about hygiene.

Liquid soap is also an inspired way to use your homemade soaps if you dislike the way the molding came out, but can't bear to toss away the product of a good recipe.

DIRECTIONS

1. In the top half of a double boiler, melt together the soap, oil, glycerin, and water.

2. When fully melted, remove from heat, add the vodka, and stir.

3. Allow soap to cool and add whatever essential oil or fragrance oil you desire.

4. Let mixture cool completely before bottling.

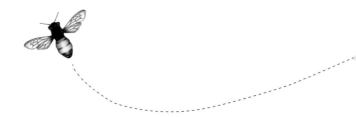

ESSENTIAL OILS AND FRAGRANCE OILS

When selecting fragrance oils for soap, make sure to buy oil that is designated as "soap safe." A fragrance that isn't soap safe for lye soap making can cause an entire batch to become clumpy or hard, or can cause the soap to curdle or discolor.

Unlike fragrance oils, which are mainly synthetic, essential oils are the natural oils from plants. As a result, they retain some of the aromatherapy benefits of the plants they were derived from, as well as contributing delightful scents to your fabrications.

When you create blends using both essential oils and fragrance oils, you need to be careful to use the proper measurements for each. Not all fragrance oils are the same, so be sure you get the manufacturer's or distributor's rate of use for each oil you include. The fragrance oils you use should be bath and body safe and approved by IFRA guidelines. Fragrance oils made for candles may irritate your skin.

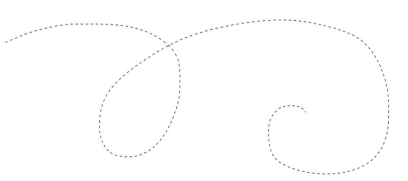

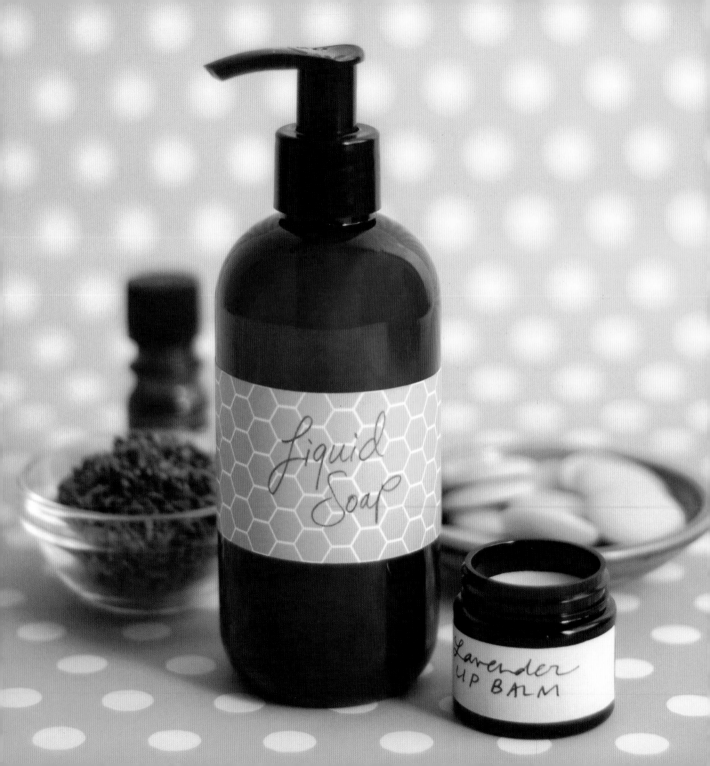

Basic Lip Balm

Hives are most active during the summer months, but the fruit of the bee's labor helps us year round. Beeswax is the most vital ingredient for making premium lip balms that can soothe chapped lips when the weather cools. The smooth surface protects your mouth from the abrasive cold air, and seals in the moisture you still have. The skin of your lips is particularly thin and must be protected from the elements, especially the drying effect of wind.

If you've been buying lip balm in stores, chances are you've paid too much for it. Balm can be made easily and inexpensively. This basic recipe yields twelve tubes or small containers of lip balm, each holding about ⅛ ounce.

DIRECTIONS

1. Combine oil with the beeswax.

2. Melt in the top half of a double boiler. Never melt beeswax directly over a flame as it could catch fire.

3. Once melted, allow the mixture to cool to 120°F. Then pour into lip balm tubes, small pots, or slider tins.

ITEMS NEEDED

- ¾ ounce (weight) beeswax
- 1½ ounces (weight) fixed oil, such as sweet almond, grape seed, coconut, or sunflower, in any combination you wish
- Double boiler
- Wax or candy thermometer
- Tubes, tins, or other containers

A NOTE ON OILS

Although you certainly can use olive oil to make lip balm, remember that it has quite a strong flavor and fragrance. If you are making flavored lip balms, like the ones you'll learn about soon, you may prefer an oil with a more neutral taste.

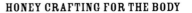

Moisturizing Lip Balm

- Double boiler
- 1½ ounces (weight) beeswax
- 1 ounce (weight) cocoa butter
- 1½ ounces (weight) shea butter
- 2 ounces (weight) coconut oil (or any combination of oils desired)
- 15 drops vitamin E oil (if using gelatin capsules, pierce with a pin and drip out oil)
- Small squirt of honey
- Wax or candy thermometer
- Tubes, tins, or other containers

Basic lip balm will insulate and protect your lips, but this craft will actively moisturize them as well. The shea and cocoa butters in this luscious lip balm produce a very creamy, rich balm that's perfect if you have a particular problem with dryness.

DIRECTIONS

1. In the top of a double boiler melt together the beeswax, cocoa butter, shea butter, coconut oil, and vitamin E oil.

2. Add a squirt of honey, stirring to incorporate as much as possible into the mixture. (What isn't absorbed into the lip balm mixture will rest on the bottom of the pot and can be ignored.)

3. Remove the mixture from heat. When it's cooled to 120°F, pour into lip balm tubes, pots, slider tins, or other containers.

4. Discard the remaining honey left at the bottom of the boiler.

Makes 36 ⅛-ounce tubes or small containers of creamy lip balm.

Cocoa Lavender Lip Balm

The floral lightness of the lavender in this delicious creation combines with the lavish chocolate flavor oil for a balm that's good enough to eat. You'll keep finding excuses to rub this along your lips. Lavender is an exceptionally versatile flower, known in aromatherapy for its soothing and relaxing properties.

DIRECTIONS

1. Combine the carrier oil with the beeswax.

2. Melt it in the top half of a double boiler. Never melt beeswax directly over a flame as it could catch fire.

3. Once melted, remove from heat.

4. Mix in the lavender essential oil and the chocolate flavor oil.

5. Allow the mixture to cool to 120°F. Then pour into lip balm tubes, small pots, or slider tins.

ITEMS NEEDED FOR THE BASIC LIP BALM

- 1½ ounces (weight) almond oil, grapeseed oil, coconut oil, or sunflower oil
- ¾ ounce (weight) beeswax
- Double boiler
- ¾₄₀ ounce (weight) lavender essential oil
- ¾₄₀ ounce (weight) chocolate flavor oil (must be oil, not extract)
- Wax or candy thermometer
- Tubes, tins, or other containers

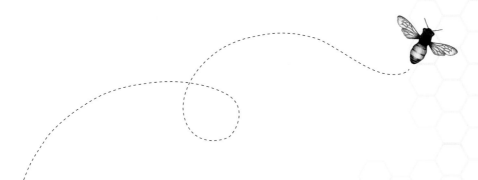

ITEMS NEEDED FOR THE MOISTURIZING LIP BALM

- Double boiler
- 1½ ounces (weight) beeswax
- 1 ounce (weight) cocoa butter
- 1½ ounces (weight) shea butter
- 2 ounces (weight) coconut oil (or any combination of oils desired)
- 15 drops vitamin E oil (if using gelatin capsules, pierce with a pin and drip out oil)
- Small squirt of honey
- ⅛ ounce (weight) lavender essential oil
- ⅛ ounce (weight) chocolate flavor oil (must be oil, not extract)
- Wax or candy thermometer
- Tubes, tins, or other containers

DIRECTIONS

1. In the top of a double boiler melt together the beeswax, cocoa butter, shea butter, coconut oil, and vitamin E oil.

2. Add a squirt of honey, stirring to incorporate as much as possible into the mixture. (What isn't absorbed into the lip balm mixture will rest on the bottom of the pot and can be ignored.)

3. Remove the mixture from heat. Mix in the lavender essential oil and the chocolate flavor oil.

4. When it's cooled to 120°F, pour into lip balm tubes, pots, slider tins, or other containers.

5. Discard the remaining honey left at the bottom of the boiler.

Makes 36 ⅛-ounce tubes or small containers of creamy lip balm.

Be sure to buy chocolate flavor oil, which is really a type of fragrance oil that has been tested for safe use on the lips. Not all fragrance oils are safe for use on the skin or lips. Be sure to read the material safety data sheet (MSDS) for each flavoring before use.

Fennel Lip Balm

In many parts of India, people chew fennel seeds to freshen their breath after a meal. This balm will give your breath a sweet scent as it protects your lips.

DIRECTIONS

1. Combine the carrier oil with the beeswax.

2. Melt it in the top half of a double boiler. Never melt beeswax directly over a flame as it could catch fire.

3. Once melted, remove from heat.

4. Mix in the fennel essential oil.

5. Allow the mixture to cool to 120°F. Then pour into lip balm tubes, small pots, or slider tins.

- 1½ ounces (weight) almond oil, grapeseed oil, coconut oil, or sunflower oil
- ¾ ounce (weight) beeswax
- Double boiler
- ¾₀ ounce (weight) fennel essential oil
- Wax or candy thermometer
- Tubes, tins, or other containers

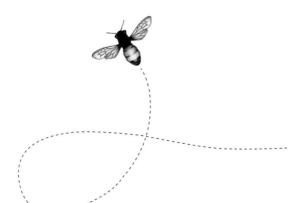

ITEMS NEEDED FOR THE MOISTURIZING LIP BALM

- Double boiler
- 1½ ounces (weight) beeswax
- 1 ounce (weight) cocoa butter
- 1½ ounces (weight) shea butter
- 2 ounces (weight) coconut oil (or any combination of oils desired)
- 15 drops vitamin E oil (if using gelatin capsules, pierce with a pin and drip out oil)
- Small squirt of honey
- ⅛ ounce (weight) fennel essential oil
- Wax or candy thermometer
- Tubes, tins, or other containers

DIRECTIONS

1. In the top of a double boiler melt together the beeswax, cocoa butter, shea butter, coconut oil, and vitamin E oil.

2. Add a squirt of honey, stirring to incorporate as much as possible into the mixture. (What isn't absorbed into the lip balm mixture will rest on the bottom of the pot and can be ignored.)

3. Remove the mixture from heat. Mix in the fennel essential oil.

4. When it's cooled to 120°F, pour into lip balm tubes, pots, slider tins, or other containers.

5. Discard the remaining honey left at the bottom of the double boiler.

Makes 36 ⅛-ounce tubes or small containers of creamy lip balm.

Mandarin Clove Lip Balm

This lip balm has a rich, heady scent that brings to mind royalty and indulgence. The cloves have a warming effect that will be most welcome if you're applying the balm on a windy winter day. The mandarin orange flavor adds a tart kick to the spicy clove—like a squeeze of juice from a fresh orange over a rich Thanksgiving pie.

DIRECTIONS

1. Combine the carrier oil with the beeswax.

2. Melt it in the top half of a double boiler. Never melt beeswax directly over a flame as it could catch fire.

3. Once melted, remove from heat.

4. Mix in the orange essential oil and the clove bud essential oil.

5. Allow the mixture to cool to 120°F. Then pour into lip balm tubes, small pots, or slider tins.

ITEMS NEEDED FOR THE BASIC LIP BALM

- 1½ ounces (weight) almond oil, grape seed oil, coconut oil, or sunflower oil
- ¾ ounce (weight) beeswax
- Double boiler
- ³⁄₄₀ ounce (weight) orange essential oil
- ³⁄₄₀ ounce (weight) clove bud essential oil
- Wax or candy thermometer
- Tubes, tins, or other containers

ITEMS NEEDED FOR THE MOISTURIZING LIP BALM

- Double boiler
- 1½ ounces (weight) beeswax
- 1 ounce (weight) cocoa butter
- 1½ ounces (weight) shea butter
- 2 ounces (weight) coconut oil (or any combination of oils desired)
- 15 drops vitamin E oil (if using gelatin capsules, pierce with a pin and drip out oil)
- Small squirt of honey
- ⅛ ounce (weight) orange essential oil
- ⅛ ounce (weight) clove bud essential oil
- Wax or candy thermometer
- Tubes, tins, or other containers

DIRECTIONS

1. In the top of a double boiler melt together the beeswax, cocoa butter, shea butter, coconut oil, and vitamin E oil.

2. Add a squirt of honey, stirring to incorporate as much as possible into the mixture. (What isn't absorbed into the lip balm mixture will rest on the bottom of the pot and can be ignored.)

3. Remove the mixture from heat. Mix in the orange essential oil and the clove bud essential oil.

4. When it's cooled to 120°F, pour into lip balm tubes, pots, slider tins, or other containers.

5. Discard the remaining honey left at the bottom of the double boiler.

Makes 36 ⅛-ounce tubes or small containers of creamy lip balm.

Basic Hand and Body Cream

Beeswax has a moisturizing effect that makes it perfect for skin care products such as creams, salves, and scrubs. It is a unique substance in that it can coat and protect, while still allowing your skin to breathe. This property makes it the ideal ingredient in body creams.

The vitamin E in these creams contains strong antioxidant properties that prevent signs of aging. This mild, scentless cream will keep your body smooth and radiant. Rub it into your skin after your normal cleaning and exfoliating regimen.

DIRECTIONS

1. Combine the oils and beeswax in the top half of a double boiler.

2. Heat just until the wax melts.

3. Remove from heat. Stir frequently while cooling.

4. Add vitamin E oil and stir.

5. Spoon cream into a clean jar.

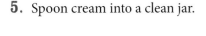

ITEMS NEEDED

- 1 cup sweet almond oil (olive oil can be substituted for any body cream if you'd prefer)

- ½ cup coconut oil

- 2 ounces (weight) beeswax

- Double boiler

- ½ teaspoon vitamin E oil

- Jar

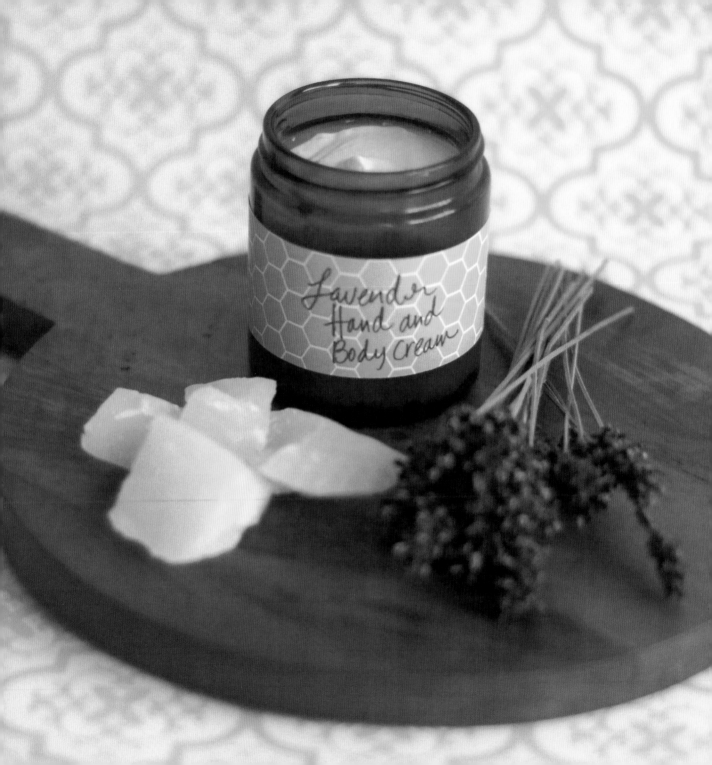

Lavender Hand and Body Cream

The elegant, gentle scent of the lavender flower will calm your nerves. Use this cream to hydrate your skin before bedtime to guarantee a restful sleep.

DIRECTIONS

1. Combine the oils and beeswax in the top half of a double boiler.

2. Heat just until the wax melts.

3. Remove from heat. Stir frequently while cooling.

4. Add vitamin E oil and lavender essential oil. Stir until fully blended.

5. Spoon cream into a clean jar.

ITEMS NEEDED

- 1 cup sweet almond oil
- ½ cup coconut oil
- 2 ounces (weight) beeswax
- Double boiler
- ½ teaspoon vitamin E oil
- 15–20 drops of lavender essential oil
- Jar

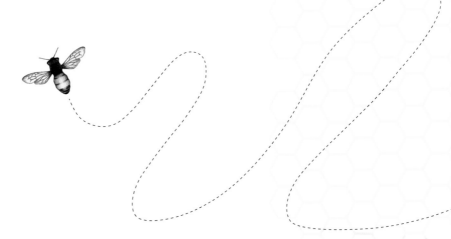

Green Tea Hand and Body Cream

ITEMS NEEDED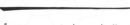

- 1 cup sweet almond oil
- ½ cup coconut oil
- 2 ounces (weight) beeswax
- Double boiler
- Wax or candy thermometer
- ½ teaspoon vitamin E oil
- 2 tablespoons powdered green tea
- Jar

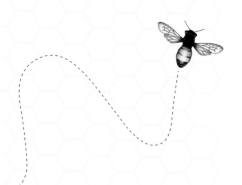

You can pick up powdered green tea at most Asian grocery shops or beauty supply outlets. It is a powerful antioxidant used throughout the world to keep the body young and healthy. Continued use of this cream, each morning and night, will keep your skin firm and bright. It also has a lovely green hue and a gentle scent that will comfort and rejuvenate.

DIRECTIONS

1. Combine the oils and wax in the top half of a double boiler.

2. Heat just until the wax melts.

3. Remove from heat. Stir frequently while cooling.

4. Once the cream has thickened to the consistency of pudding and is below 120°F, add vitamin E oil and powdered green tea. Stir until fully blended.

5. Spoon cream into a clean jar. The cream will continue to thicken as it cools.

Lemon Mint Hand and Body Cream

The lemon in this recipe acts as an astringent, making this a perfect cream for oily skin. The mint will cool your skin after a day outside in the sun.

DIRECTIONS

1. Combine the almond and coconut oils and wax in the top half of a double boiler.

2. Heat just until the wax melts.

3. Remove from heat. Stir frequently while cooling.

4. Add vitamin E oil, lemon essential oil, and peppermint essential oil. Stir until fully blended.

5. Spoon cream into a clean jar.

ITEMS NEEDED

- 1 cup sweet almond oil
- ½ cup coconut oil
- 2 ounces (weight) beeswax
- Double boiler
- ½ teaspoon vitamin E oil
- 15 drops of lemon essential oil
- 5 drops of peppermint essential oil
- Jar

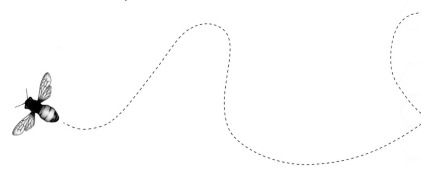

Basic Skin Scrub

- 26-ounce container of sea salt crystals (*sel de mer*)

- 4 ounces (weight) oil—can be any combination of oils (olive, coconut, sweet almond, sunflower, avocado, etc.)

- 3 ounces (weight) liquid castile soap (instructions found earlier in this section). If you have not prepared your own, any gentle liquid soap or unscented body wash will do.

- ¼ cup honey

- Large bowl

- Jars

Scrubs play an important part in keeping your skin healthy. The dead skin cells on the surface of your back, hands, and legs can clog pores, leading to blemishes or dryness. Scrubs let you gently exfoliate your skin, clearing away the old cells to reveal the glowing skin underneath. This is an excellent basic recipe if you're bothered by scented bath products. Note that salt scrubs can be too strong for the sensitive skin on your face. Use these scrubs for the rest of your body, instead. The Sugar Facial Scrub with Honey, which you'll find later in this chapter, is a gentler scrub that's perfect for your cheeks and forehead.

DIRECTIONS

1. Mix all of the ingredients together in a large bowl.

2. Once thoroughly blended, pack into decorative or canning jars.

3. Refrigerate.

HOW TO USE A SCRUB

1. Rinse face with warm water.
2. Spoon out a dollop of scrub into your hand, or onto a washcloth.
3. Gently scrub face using a circular motion, taking care to avoid the delicate skin around the eyes.
4. Splash off using generous amounts of warm water.
5. Follow with your favorite moisturizer.

Peppermint and Orange Scrub

Mint and citrus are a rousing combination in this scrub. Both aromas have a stimulating effect that keeps you awake and alert. Use this scrub first thing in the morning for a refreshing feeling that will last all day.

DIRECTIONS

1. In a large bowl, mix together the essential oils and seeds.

2. Mix in the salt crystals, oil, liquid soap, and honey.

3. Once thoroughly blended, pack into decorative or canning jars.

4. Refrigerate.

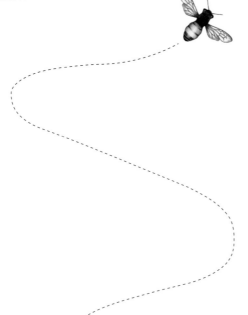

- Large bowl
- ½ teaspoon peppermint essential oil
- 1 teaspoon orange essential oil
- 2 teaspoons dried raspberry seeds or poppy seeds
- 26-ounce container of sea salt crystals (*sel de mer*)
- 4 ounces (weight) oil—can be any combination of oils (olive, coconut, sweet almond, sunflower, avocado, etc.)
- 3 ounces (weight) liquid castile soap (instructions found earlier in this section). If you have not prepared your own, any gentle liquid soap or unscented body wash will do.
- ¼ cup honey
- Jars

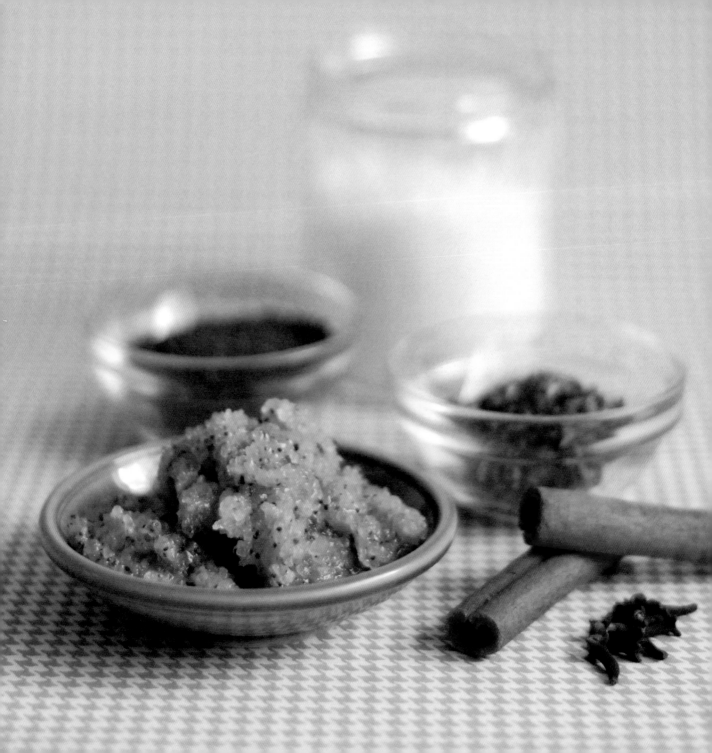

Chai Tea Body Scrub

Masala chai is a spicy black tea. Common in India, it has a loyal worldwide following of enthusiasts who love its exotic taste and invigorating effect. The combination of chai, cloves, and cinnamon produces a warming scrub that will activate and excite new cells as it gently removes dead skin.

DIRECTIONS

1. Open the tea bags and remove the contents. Dispose of the empty bags.

2. Mix the contents of the tea bags with the cinnamon, cloves, cardamom, and poppy seeds.

3. Mix in the salt crystals, oil, liquid soap, and honey.

4. Once thoroughly blended, pack into decorative or canning jars.

5. Refrigerate.

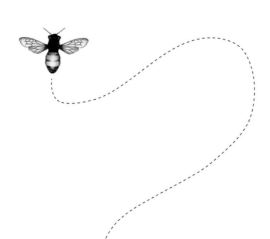

ITEMS NEEDED

- Large bowl
- 2 masala chai tea bags
- ¼ teaspoon ground cinnamon
- ¼ teaspoon ground cloves
- ¼ teaspoon ground cardamom
- 2 teaspoons poppy seeds
- 26-ounce container of sea salt crystals (*sel de mer*)
- 4 ounces (weight) oil—can be any combination of oils (olive, coconut, sweet almond, sunflower, avocado, etc.)
- 3 ounces (weight) liquid castile soap (instructions found earlier in this section). If you have not prepared your own, any gentle liquid soap or unscented body wash will do.
- ¼ cup honey
- Jars

Sugar Facial Scrub with Honey

ITEMS NEEDED

- Large bowl
- 1 cup granulated sugar
- 1 cup honey
- 2 tablespoons olive oil
- 2–3 drops of your favorite essential oil
- Jar

This simple, rejuvenating facial scrub harnesses the full healing power of honey. Honey has properties that can kill harmful bacteria that live on your skin, and cause blemishes and infections. It's also rich with vitamin B_6 that can prevent your skin from become scaly and irritated.

DIRECTIONS

1. In a large bowl, briskly mix together the sugar, honey, and oils until fully blended.

2. Refrigerate in a tightly covered jar.

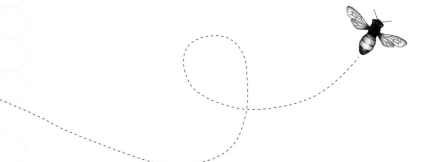

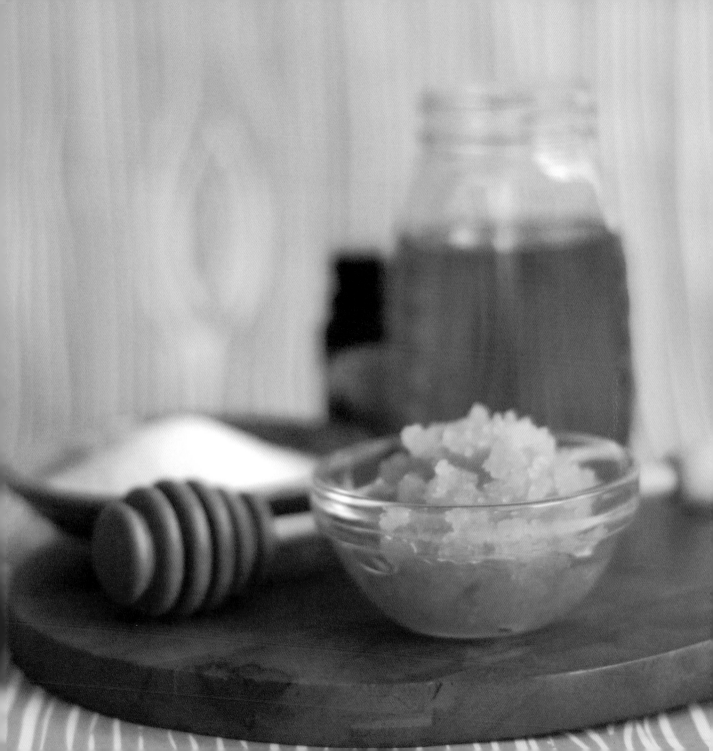

Herbal Healing Salve

ITEMS NEEDED

- 2 ounces (weight) beeswax
- 8 ounces (weight) shea butter
- 3 ounces (weight) sweet almond oil
- 1 ounce (weight) cocoa butter
- ½ ounce (weight) coconut oil
- 20 drops tea tree oil
- 20 drops calendula oil
- 5 drops orange oil
- 15 drops lavender oil
- 12 drops rosemary oil
- 8 drops cinnamon oil
- 15 drops atlas cedar oil
- Double boiler
- Small pots or jars

This salve is perfect for overly dry, rough, or scaly skin. A light coating should be rubbed onto the washed and dried area three or four times a day until symptoms ease. Never apply salve to an open wound, or to the eyes. To test for allergy, try applying a small amount to the back of the neck or inside of the elbow and see if there is a negative reaction. If refrigerated, the salves in this book will last up to one year.

DIRECTIONS

1. Combine all the ingredients in the top half of a double boiler.

2. Heat the ingredients just until the beeswax melts, then remove from heat.

3. Pour into small pots or jars, while the mixture is still warm.

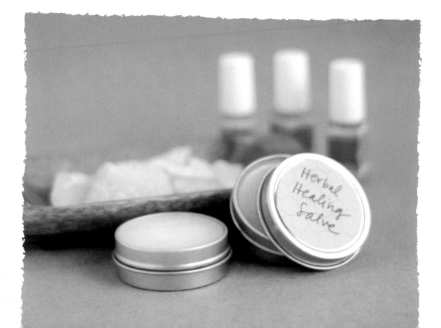

Sunburn Salve

Here's a natural way to soothe the red-hot pain, followed by peeling and itching, that too much sun can inflict upon your skin. Use this salve as soon as you realize you've been burned. The aloe vera will help ease the redness and the hurt. The beeswax, shea butter, cocoa butter, and oils will moisturize your sun-dried skin. Bring a tin with you on your next jaunt at the beach.

DIRECTIONS

1. Combine all the ingredients in the top half of a double boiler.

2. Heat the ingredients just until the beeswax melts, then remove from heat.

3. Pour into small pots or jars, while the mixture is still warm.

- 2 ounces (weight) beeswax
- 8 ounces (weight) shea butter
- 3 ounces (weight) sweet almond oil
- 1 ounce (weight) cocoa butter
- ½ ounce (weight) coconut oil
- ½ cup aloe vera gel
- 20 drops lavender essential oil
- 20 drops peppermint essential oil
- Double boiler
- Small pots or jars

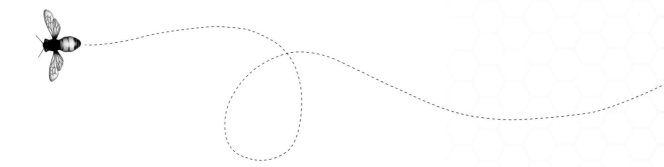

Vapor Salve

ITEMS NEEDED

- 2 ounces (weight) beeswax
- 8 ounces (weight)shea butter
- 3 ounces (weight) sweet almond oil
- 1 ounce (weight) cocoa butter
- ½ ounce (weight) coconut oil
- 20 drops eucalyptus essential oil
- 20 drops peppermint essential oil
- Double boiler
- Small pots or jars

The eucalyptus and peppermint in this ointment will soothe a rasping cough. Rub the cream on your chest and feel relief spread all over as you begin to breathe easy.

DIRECTIONS

1. Combine all the ingredients in the top half of a double boiler.

2. Heat the ingredients just until the beeswax melts, then remove from heat.

3. Pour into small pots or jars, while the mixture is still warm.

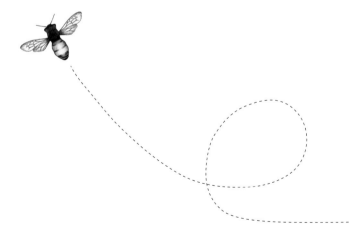

Heart-Healthy Hawthorn Syrup

This syrup incorporates hawthorn berries, which are rich in antioxidants and have proven cardiovascular benefits. If the berries have seeds in them, soak and press them through a sieve to remove the seeds before using. If properly stored, the syrups in this book will last for several weeks.

DIRECTIONS

1. Put the berries into a pan with just enough apple juice to cover them. Simmer over low heat for 15 minutes. Remove from heat and let stand overnight.

2. Season with honey, ginger, and cinnamon to taste.

3. Return to heat, add enough apple juice to create a syrupy consistency, and heat through.

4. Remove from heat, let cool, and transfer to glass bottles. Store in the refrigerator.

ITEMS NEEDED

- A handful of dried seedless hawthorn berries
- Saucepan
- Apple juice (enough to cover berries in pan)
- Honey to taste
- Ginger to taste, grated or powdered
- Cinnamon to taste
- Glass bottles

DOSAGE

Adults should take ½–1 teaspoon three times a day to keep their hearts healthy.

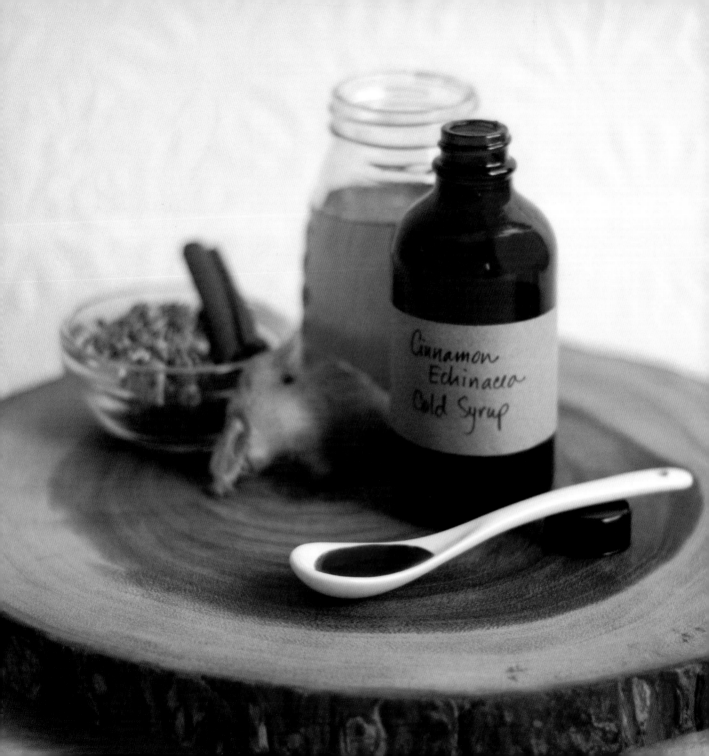

Cinnamon Echinacea Cold Syrup

You've heard that a spoonful of sugar helps the medicine go down, but honey is even better. This one is useful to have on hand during flu season. Some studies have shown that echinacea boosts your immune system. Cinnamon and ginger have long been home remedies for the sniffles. And anyone who's sipped hot tea with honey for a sore throat knows how soothing it can be.

DIRECTIONS

1. Add 2 ounces (about 8 tablespoons) of the herb mixture to a quart of cold water. Bring to a boil, then simmer until the liquid is reduced by half (leave the lid slightly ajar).

2. Strain the herbs from the liquid and discard, then pour the liquid back into the pot.

3. Add 1 cup of honey and heat the mixture through.

4. Remove from heat, let cool, and transfer to glass bottles. Store in the refrigerator.

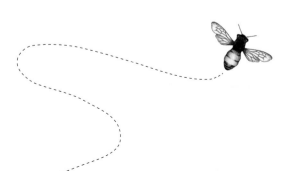

ITEMS NEEDED

- 1 part dried echinacea root
- 1 part cinnamon bark
- ½ part fresh gingerroot, grated or chopped
- 1 quart water
- Pot with lid
- 1 cup honey
- Glass bottles

DOSAGE

Adults should take ½–1 teaspoon three times a day for chronic conditions. When treating an acute problem, take ¼–½ teaspoon every 30–60 minutes, until symptoms improve. Children and seniors should be given smaller doses.

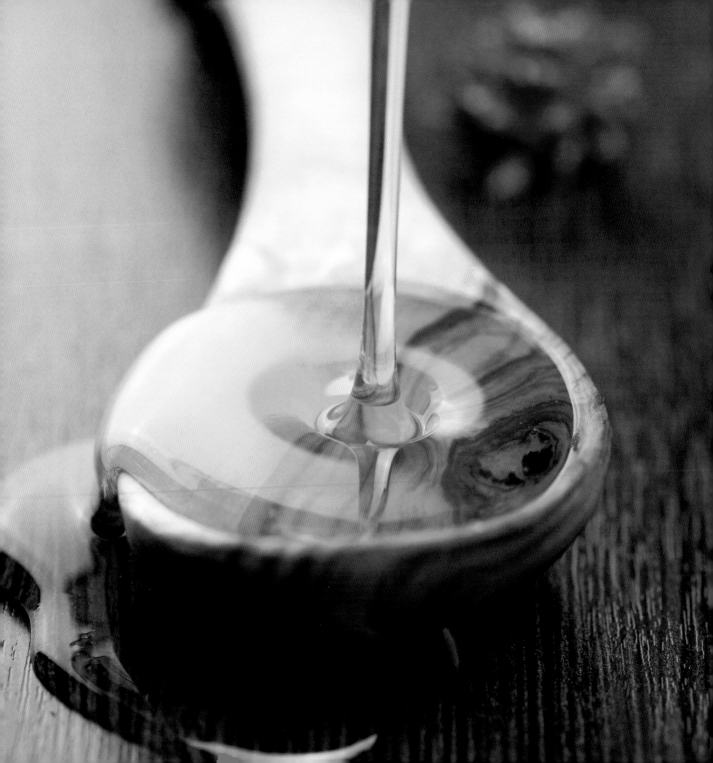

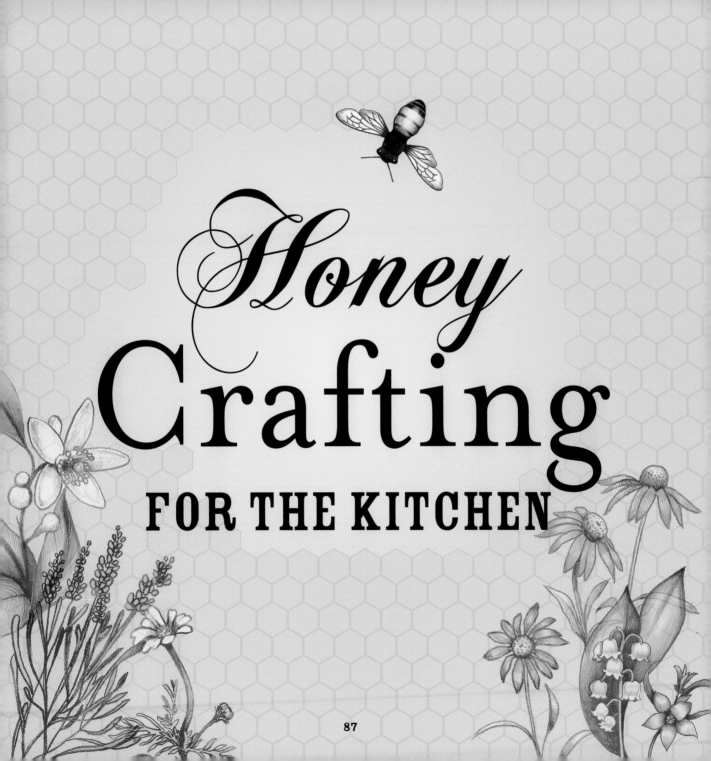

Honey Crafting

FOR THE KITCHEN

Introduction

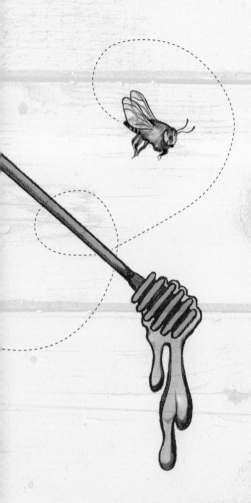

Think back to your first memory of honey. It was probably not in a soap or a cream. It was probably not in the scent from a candle. Most likely, your first memory of honey was the taste.

You remember the thickness of the syrup rolling from your lips onto your tongue, coating the sides of your throat in a soothing veneer as you swallowed. You remember the sweetness, so much richer and more interesting than sugar—a sweetness that spoke of industrious, buzzing bees and teeming hives.

On its own, without any sort of additive or embellishment, honey is a mouthwatering substance. But one of the most wondrous things about honey is what it can do when it's combined with other foods and flavors. It transforms drab dishes into festive centerpieces. It adds complexity and delight to everything it touches.

In this section, you'll learn how to infuse honeys with flavors such as cinnamon and garlic. This is honey crafting for the kitchen in its purest form—the substance you create can be used as natural honey can. Try these new infusions on their own, as suggested, or in some of the later recipes for a tantalizing twist.

Some of the recipes offered here use the sweetness of honey to accentuate and improve savory meals. Meat and fowl, such as goose, steak, and turkey, will shine, taking on new dimensions with the addition of the hive's syrup. Vegetables and nuts will spring to life when cooked or coated with a good local honey.

And, of course, you'll learn to make luscious desserts that'll have you counting the moments until your main course is over. Honey-swirled ice creams and honey-soaked pastries will have you scraping your serving plate and wishing for more. Explore and experiment with different types of honey for a new delicious dish every time.

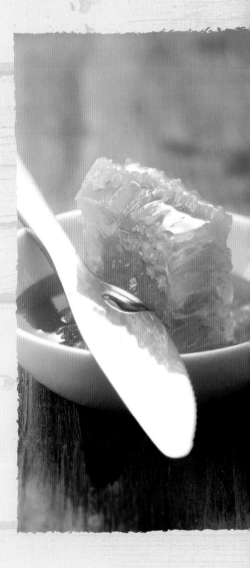

WARNING

Never feed honey to a child under one year of age as some toxins in honey can make infants sick. Talk to your physician about the proper time to introduce your child to the taste of the hive.

Infusions

Infusing honey with different and exotic flavors is an excellent way to enjoy this versatile and unique substance. By infusing honey, you're enhancing the original flavor without losing any of the properties that make it so beneficial and appealing. Store the infused honeys in jars or squeeze bottles. Make your own labels for lovely gifts that friends and family will enjoy.

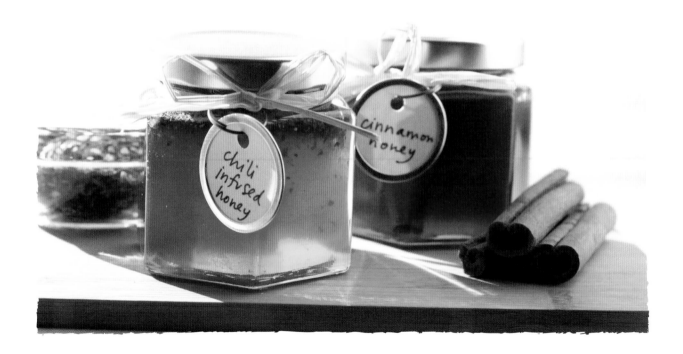

Cinnamon Honey

Cinnamon honey is a delicious and healthy alternative to pancake syrup. Try it on baked goods, pastries, and French toast. It makes tea taste wonderful, too!

DIRECTIONS

1. Heat the honey in the top of a double boiler to 180°F. Heating to this temperature aids in mixing, and also will prevent the honey from later forming crystals around the cinnamon particles.

2. Add 2 tablespoons ground cinnamon and stir until completely blended.

3. Pour into a wide-mouth jar or squeeze bottle, and set the mixture aside to infuse for 2 or 3 days.

- 2 cups honey
- 2 tablespoons ground cinnamon

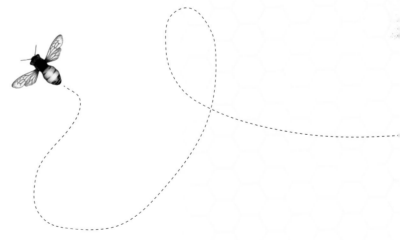

Chili-Infused Honey

INGREDIENTS

- 2 cups honey
- ¼ teaspoon citric acid granules (can be purchased at your local health foods store) to maintain acid pH and prevent botulism
- ½ cup finely chopped fresh chili peppers, washed and dried, or 4 tablespoons dried chili pepper flakes

Try chili-infused honey on crackers with soft cheeses, such as brie. Brush it on chicken after barbecuing.

DIRECTIONS

1. Heat honey in the top of a double boiler to 180°F.

2. Add citric acid and stir until completely blended. Mix in chilies. Carefully monitoring temperature, continue to heat the mixture at 180°F for half an hour.

3. Pour into a wide-mouth jar or squeeze bottles, cover, and set the mixture aside to cool and continue infusing for 2 or 3 days.

You can make chili-infused honey without heating the honey. Mix ingredients in a large jar, cover tightly, and allow to sit away from sunlight for up to 3 weeks for best flavor.

Ginger-Infused Honey

Try ginger-infused honey on grilled salmon or in tea. Mix two tablespoons of infused honey into soda water for homemade ginger ale.

DIRECTIONS

1. Heat honey in the top of a double boiler to 180°F.

2. Add citric acid and stir until completely blended. Mix in ginger.

3. Carefully monitoring temperature, continue to heat the mixture at 180°F for half an hour.

4. Pour into a wide-mouth jar or squeeze bottles, cover, and set the mixture aside to cool and continue infusing for 2 or 3 days.

You can make ginger-infused honey without heating the honey. Mix ingredients in a large jar, cover tightly, and allow to sit away from sunlight for up to 3 weeks for best flavor.

INGREDIENTS

- 2 cups honey
- ¼ teaspoon citric acid granules (can be purchased at your local health foods store) to maintain acid pH and prevent botulism
- ½ cup finely chopped peeled fresh ginger, washed and dried

SUBSTITUTIONS

If you don't have any fresh ginger on hand, substitute either 2 tablespoons chopped dried ginger or 1 tablespoon ginger powder.

Garlic-Infused Honey

INGREDIENTS

- 2 cups honey
- ¼ teaspoon citric acid granules (can be purchased at your local health foods store) to maintain acid pH and prevent botulism
- ½ cup finely chopped fresh peeled garlic, washed

Garlic honey makes an interesting and surprisingly delicious dessert topping to serve over vanilla ice cream. Garlic honey has also been used for centuries as a cold and flu remedy—eat a spoonful every few hours until symptoms lessen.

DIRECTIONS

1. Heat honey in the top of a double boiler to 180°F.

2. Add citric acid and stir until completely blended.

3. Mix in garlic.

4. Carefully monitoring temperature, continue to heat the mixture at 180°F for half an hour.

5. Pour into a wide-mouth jar or squeeze bottles, cover, and set the mixture aside to cool and continue infusing for 2 or 3 days.

You can make garlic-infused honey without heating the honey. Mix ingredients in a large jar, cover tightly, and allow to sit away from sunlight for up to 3 weeks for best flavor.

Savory

Honey and ham have long been the combination of choice when using the bees' elixir for savory fare. Without that delightful brown coat, holiday hams would be drab and pink indeed. But gourmets who crave honey in meals will discover many other options that will make your eyes widen and your mouths water.

Honey provides the perfect texture for glazing meats. It cuts the tang of vinegar for an excellent salad dressing or marinade. It gives vegetables such as carrots and beets entirely new and different textures and tastes. By exploring the recipes in this section, you'll be amazed by what honey can bring to the dinner table, hors d'oeuvre plate, and leisurely lunch.

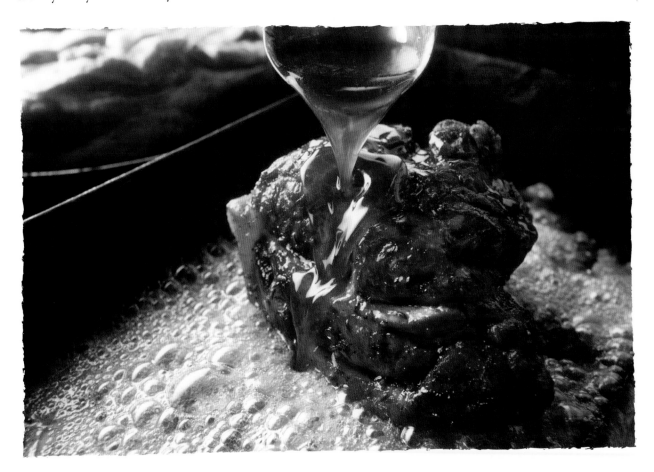

Honey-Orange Beets

- 6 medium-sized fresh beets
- 1 teaspoon grated orange zest
- 2 tablespoons orange juice
- 2 teaspoons butter
- 1 teaspoon honey
- ¼ teaspoon ground ginger
- Salt and freshly ground pepper to taste

This light, delectable vegetable dish makes a fine addition to a summer meal. If you're using beets with the greens still attached, remove them, dress them in lemon and olive oil, and use them as a bed for the dish. It will look as wonderful on the plate as it tastes.

DIRECTIONS

1. In a pot of boiling water, cook beets for 40 minutes or until tender.

2. Drain beets and let cool slightly. Slip off skins and slice.

3. In a saucepan, heat the orange zest, orange juice, butter, honey, and ginger over low heat until the butter melts.

4. Add the beets, and toss to coat. Season with salt and pepper.

Serves 4

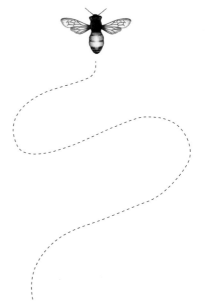

Honey-Glazed Filet Mignon

Taking a bite of this dish is like sliding headfirst into the lap of luxury. Filet mignon is the most expensive cut of meat, and its succulent taste and texture combined with a honey glaze will produce a meal that's hard to forget.

DIRECTIONS

1. Season steaks with salt and pepper.

2. Heat a large nonstick skillet over medium heat and add olive oil. Add steaks to pan and cook for 4 minutes, until easy to turn. Carefully turn steaks and cook for 3–5 minutes until desired doneness. Remove from pan and cover with foil to keep warm.

3. Add garlic and shallots to pan; turn heat to medium high. Cook and stir to loosen pan drippings. Add honey and wine and bring to a boil. Boil for a few minutes to reduce sauce. Return steaks to pan and cook for 1 minute to heat through, spooning sauce over steaks. Serve immediately.

Serves 6

INGREDIENTS

- 6 (4-ounce) filet mignon steaks
- ½ teaspoon salt
- ⅛ teaspoon pepper
- 1 tablespoon olive oil
- 3 cloves garlic, minced
- 2 shallots, minced
- 3 tablespoons honey
- ¼ cup dry red wine

Glazed Turnips

INGREDIENTS

- 2 pounds turnips
- 2 tablespoons butter
- ¼ cup honey
- ¼ teaspoon ground ginger
- Salt and freshly ground pepper to taste

If you've tried turnips before and found them bland, they were probably cooked incorrectly. Take care not to overcook them, and the honey and ginger will do the rest.

DIRECTIONS

1. Peel turnips and cut into ½-inch thick, quarter-sized slices.

2. In a pot of boiling water, cook turnips for 8 minutes or just until tender; drain.

3. Stir in butter and cook over high heat, shaking pan often, until vegetables are coated with butter. Stir in honey, ginger, and salt and pepper to taste. Cook, stirring often, for 1 minute or until glazed. Serve immediately.

Serves 4

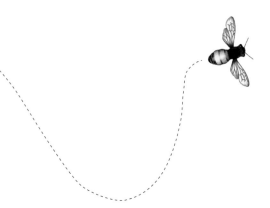

Soy and Honey Roasted Black Cod

Black cod is a great substitute for Chilean sea bass, which is being fished to extinction. The mixture of soy sauce and honey is an exciting combination that will tempt those with a taste for adventure.

DIRECTIONS

1. Boil the string beans in salted water until they are tender but still crisp, about 5 minutes. Cool them in ice water and drain well. Toss the beans with the sesame seeds, sesame oil, and a bit of salt and pepper. Set aside.

2. Mix together the soy sauce, oil, and honey. Coat the cod in the mixture and let it marinate for about 2 hours (an hour on each side) in the refrigerator.

3. Preheat oven to 425°F.

4. Place the fish in a small, ovenproof sauté pan. Roast in the oven for about 12 minutes or until the fish has browned well on top and is piping hot in the middle. Serve with the sesame string beans on a large plate.

INGREDIENTS

- 2 cups trimmed string beans
- 1 tablespoon toasted sesame seeds
- 1 tablespoon sesame oil
- Salt and pepper, to taste
- 3 tablespoons soy sauce
- 1 tablespoon vegetable oil
- 3 tablespoons honey
- 2 (6-ounce) black cod fillets

Spiced Mixed Nuts

- ¼ cup honey
- 1 tablespoon red pepper flakes
- 2 tablespoons olive oil
- 1 teaspoon kosher salt
- ½ teaspoon cayenne pepper
- 3 cups mixed nuts

This is a great recipe for a party. The nuts are easy to make in quantity and can be stored in an airtight container. However, many people have allergies to nuts, so be sure to check with your guests ahead of time if you choose to make this dish.

DIRECTIONS

1. Preheat oven to 300°F.

2. Line a baking sheet with parchment paper and lightly oil the paper. Set the baking sheet aside.

3. Place all the ingredients except the mixed nuts in a medium-sized nonstick skillet over medium heat. Cook uncovered, stirring frequently, until the mixture reaches a syrup consistency, about 2–3 minutes.

4. Add the nuts and gently fold them into the syrup mixture until evenly coated. Use a rubber spatula to make the mixing easier and take care not to break up the nuts.

5. Transfer the nuts to the prepared baking sheet and spread out in an even layer. Bake for about 20 minutes, stirring and turning the nuts every 6–8 minutes. Be very watchful during the last half of baking, as the nuts can burn quickly. Serve warm or at room temperature.

Serves 12

Not all nuts are the same. If you're watching your calories, pistachios and cashews are great nuts for you to munch on. Almonds have lots of protein, and low saturated fat, making them a smart snacking choice as well. Walnuts have high levels of the healthy omega-3 fatty acids. Of course, sometimes you'll just want to eat the nuts that are the most delicious.

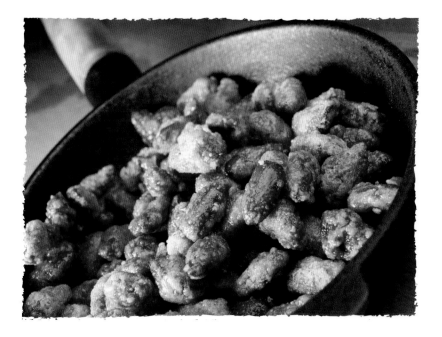

Honey Mustard Pork Chops

- 2 tablespoons olive oil
- 2 (8-ounce) center-cut, bone-in pork chops
- Salt and pepper, to taste
- 2 tablespoons butter
- 2 Granny Smith apples, peeled, cored, and cut into 8 wedges each
- 4 tablespoons Dijon mustard
- 3 tablespoons honey

You've probably seen illustrations or even photographs of people serving a pig with an apple in its mouth. That's because the tenderness of pork pairs particularly well with sweet flavors, such as fruit and honey. Get that same taste here, but without feeding an apple to a boar.

DIRECTIONS

1. Preheat oven to 450°F. Heat the olive oil in a heavy skillet on medium high.

2. Season the pork chops with salt and pepper, and brown well, about 2 minutes per side.

3. Wipe out the pan and add the butter. Heat on medium until it stops bubbling, and add the apples. Season with salt and pepper, and sauté for about 5 minutes or until the apples soften slightly and brown. Remove the apples from the pan and keep warm.

4. Mix together the mustard and honey, and rub on top of the pork chops. Place the chops on a baking sheet, and roast for 6 minutes or until the tops are glazed and the center reaches 155°F. Let rest for a few minutes, and serve with the apples on top of the chops.

Classic Steakhouse Salad

One of the most common ways to incorporate honey into savory cooking is in the form of dressings or marinades. This vinaigrette was developed for Eric Rifkin, co-owner and executive chef of the Crazy Dog Restaurant in Long Island. It has become his house dressing and guests buy quarts of it to take home. Make extra.

DIRECTIONS

1. Make the vinaigrette by combining the vinegar, honey, mustard, and garlic in a food processor. With the processor running, slowly add the oil in a thin stream until it is emulsified and the dressing has a light-brown color.

2. Arrange the tomato and onion in alternating slices in the centers of two salad plates. Season with salt and pepper.

3. Top with the crumbled blue cheese and a generous amount of the vinaigrette.

INGREDIENTS

- 1 cup balsamic vinegar
- ½ cup honey
- 2 tablespoons Dijon mustard
- 2 garlic cloves, smashed
- 3 cups canola oil
- 1 large or 2 small beefsteak tomatoes, cored and sliced into ¼-inch-thick rounds
- 1 large Vidalia onion, sliced into ¼-inch-thick rounds
- Salt and pepper, to taste
- ½ cup crumbled blue cheese

Creamy Cabbage Spring Rolls

INGREDIENTS

- Peanut oil, as needed
- 1 tablespoon minced fresh gingerroot
- 2 garlic cloves, smashed
- 3 scallions, thinly sliced
- 1 small head Napa cabbage, thinly sliced
- 2 tablespoons soy sauce
- 2 teaspoons sesame oil
- 1 teaspoon granulated sugar
- 4 spring roll wrappers
- 3 tablespoons honey
- 1 tablespoon Chinese chili paste or sambal

Napa cabbage is essential to this dish. Only this soft and supple cabbage will provide the silky, almost creamy texture for the filling in these crispy spring rolls. The honey in the dipping sauce will bring these enchanting hors d'oeuvres to life.

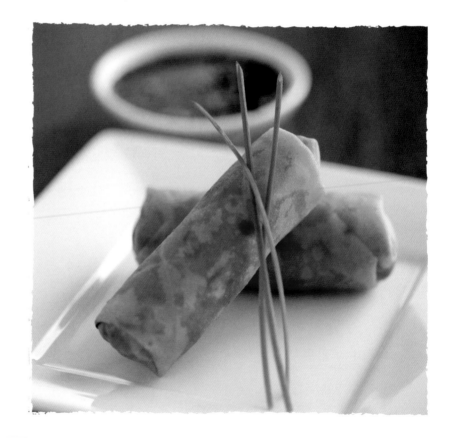

DIRECTIONS

1. In a large, heavy sauté pan or wok, heat 3 tablespoons of the peanut oil until barely smoking. Add the ginger, garlic, and scallions, and sauté for 1 minute.

2. Add the cabbage and stir-fry for about 3 minutes or until the cabbage is well wilted. Add the soy sauce, sesame oil, and sugar. Continue cooking for 1 minute. Transfer the cabbage to a colander and let drain for 10 minutes. Cool until it is comfortable to handle.

3. Place about 2 tablespoons of the cabbage in the center of each spring roll wrapper. Tuck in the sides of the wrapper and roll up like a burrito. Seal the edge with a drop of water.

4. In a pot, heat about 1 inch of the peanut oil to 350°F. Fry the spring rolls for about 2 minutes or until very crispy. Drain on paper towels.

5. Mix together the honey and chili paste and serve on the side to dip.

Goose Braised with Citrus and Honey

INGREDIENTS

- 2 yellow onions
- 1 carrot
- 1 stalk celery
- 1 grapefruit
- 2 oranges
- 1 lemon
- 1 lime
- 1 tablespoon olive oil
- 3-pound goose
- ½ cup port wine
- ¼ cup honey
- 2 cups beef stock

Goose can have a very gamey flavor. The tartness of the orange and lemon cut through that heavy taste, lightening the dish.

DIRECTIONS

1. Preheat oven to 350°F.

2. Cut the onions into wedges. Peel and cut the carrot into quarters. Roughly chop the celery. Quarter the grapefruit, oranges, lemon, and lime (leave the peels on).

3. Heat the oil to medium-high temperature in a large Dutch oven. Sear the goose on all sides. Add the vegetables and fruit; cook for 5 minutes, stirring constantly. Add the wine and reduce by half, then add the honey and stock. When the liquid begins to boil, cover and braise in the oven for 3–4 hours.

4. Serve the cooking liquid (which will thicken as it cooks) as a sauce accompanying the goose.

Serves 6

Honey Gorgonzola Toasts

Gorgonzola is a kind of blue cheese, and it has a very distinct taste and smell. Some people love it instantly, and others need to get used to its pungency. The honey and the cream allow eaters to have a gentle introduction to this strong, but worthwhile cheese. Offer these creamy toasts as an appetizer before a casual dinner party or serve them as an accompaniment to a salad of baby mixed greens.

DIRECTIONS

1. Preheat oven to 350°F. Slice the baguette into ¼-inch rounds and lay them out on an ungreased cookie sheet. Toast them in the oven for about 5 minutes, then turn them over and toast the other side. Remove from oven and set aside.

2. In a bowl, combine Gorgonzola and heavy cream and mix well to a spreadable consistency. Add more cream if necessary.

3. Spread each toast round with 1 tablespoon of the Gorgonzola mixture, and then drizzle honey on top of them.

4. Turn the oven to "broil" and broil the toasts just until they are browned, about 3 minutes.

Serves 4

INGREDIENTS

- 1 baguette loaf French bread
- 8 ounces Gorgonzola cheese
- 2 tablespoons heavy cream
- ¼ cup honey

Honey Mustard Turkey Tenderloins

INGREDIENTS

- 3¾ pounds turkey tenderloins
- 2 tablespoons olive oil
- ⅓ cup Dijon mustard
- ¼ cup honey
- ½ teaspoon salt
- ¼ teaspoon pepper
- ¼ cup yogurt
- 2 cups soft whole wheat bread crumbs
- ¼ cup grated Parmesan cheese
- 1 teaspoon dried thyme leaves

Honey and mustard are such a popular combination that they've become a sauce in their own right. It's truly the best of both worlds. The spiciness of the mustard is mellowed by the syrup of the honey. The honey is thinned by the mustard, to create a marinade that is flavorful, but not syrupy.

DIRECTIONS

1. Cut turkey tenderloins in half crosswise and place in shallow baking dish. In small bowl, combine olive oil, mustard, honey, salt, pepper, and yogurt and pour over turkey. Cover and marinate in refrigerator for 18–24 hours.

2. When ready to eat, preheat oven to 325°F. Combine bread crumbs, cheese, and thyme on a plate. Remove turkey from marinade and shake off excess. Roll turkey in bread-crumb mixture to coat. Place on cookie sheet.

3. Bake for 20 minutes, then carefully turn turkey over and bake for 20–30 minutes longer, until juices run clear. Serve immediately.

Serves 6

Melted Cheese Rolls

These rolls must be served warm, while the cheese is still melted and soft. The creamy combination of the honey and the cheddar makes for dripping, magnificent dinner rolls—you'll lick your fingers after eating.

DIRECTIONS

1. In medium saucepan, combine juice, water, and milk; bring to a boil. Stir in cornmeal; cook over medium heat, stirring constantly, until mixture thickens. Remove from heat and stir in honey and 2 tablespoons of butter. Let cool for 30 minutes.

2. In large bowl, combine whole wheat flour, bread flour, ½ cup all-purpose flour, salt, and yeast; mix well. Add orange juice mixture; beat for 2 minutes.

3. Gradually add enough remaining all-purpose flour to form a stiff dough. Knead dough on lightly floured surface until smooth and elastic, about 8–9 minutes. Place in a greased bowl, turning to grease top.

4. Cover and let rise until doubled, about 1 hour. Punch down dough and divide into three pieces. Knead ⅓ of the cheese cubes into each section of dough. Divide each third into twelve pieces; roll into smooth balls.

5. Place balls on greased cookie sheets about 2 inches apart. Cover and let rise until doubled, about 30–40 minutes. Preheat oven to 350°F. Bake rolls for 20–30 minutes until deep golden brown. Brush with the 2 tablespoons melted butter and remove to wire racks to cool; serve warm.

Makes 36 rolls

INGREDIENTS

- ½ cup orange juice
- 1 cup water
- ½ cup skim milk
- ½ cup cornmeal
- ½ cup honey
- 2 tablespoons butter
- 2 cups whole wheat flour
- 1 cup bread flour
- 2–3 cups all-purpose flour
- 1½ teaspoons salt
- 1¼-ounce package active dry yeast
- 2½ cups diced sharp cheddar cheese
- 2 tablespoons butter, melted

Lemon-Honey Shrimp with Prosciutto

INGREDIENTS

- 1¼ pounds shrimp (21–25 count), peeled and deveined
- 3 ounces prosciutto, very thinly sliced
- 3 tablespoons olive oil
- Freshly cracked black pepper
- ½ cup vegetable or chicken stock
- 2 tablespoons lemon juice
- 1 tablespoon honey
- Salt, to taste

Both shrimp and lemon share a bright, light taste. The honey and the salty prosciutto contrast with that, giving this seafood dish a welcome depth.

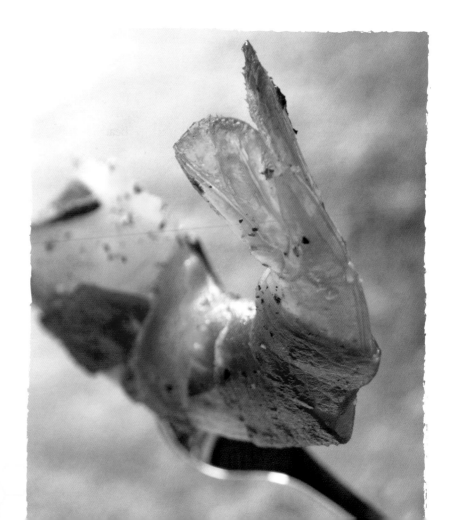

DIRECTIONS

1. Pat the shrimp dry with paper towels. Cut the prosciutto into strips about 1½ inches wide and 2½–3 inches long. Wrap a strip of prosciutto around the center of each shrimp, pressing lightly to seal.

2. Heat the oil in a large nonstick skillet over medium-high heat. Add the shrimp and cook, turning once, until the shrimp start to turn pink and the prosciutto starts to crisp, about 4–5 minutes. Season with pepper. Transfer the shrimp to a plate and tent with tinfoil to keep warm.

3. Add the stock, lemon juice, and honey to the pan and bring to a simmer. Add the shrimp and any accumulated juices to the pan and stir to coat the shrimp evenly, being careful not to damage the prosciutto wrapping. Heat through, about 1–2 minutes. Season to taste with salt and pepper, and serve hot.

Sweet and Spicy Carrots

INGREDIENTS

- 2 16-ounce packages baby carrots
- 1 cup orange juice
- 2 tablespoons butter
- ¼ cup honey
- 2 tablespoons brown sugar
- ½ cup apricot preserves
- 3 tablespoons Dijon mustard
- ¼ teaspoon salt
- ⅛ teaspoon white pepper

Serve this warm, inviting side dish when the weather gets cooler. The carrots cook to become very tender and soft—their consistency will have very little in common with raw carrot sticks.

DIRECTIONS

1. In large saucepan, combine carrots and orange juice. Bring to a boil over high heat. Cover pan, reduce heat to low, and simmer for 8–10 minutes until carrots are crisp-tender. Drain, reserving ¼ cup of the liquid.

2. Combine cooked carrots, reserved juice, and remaining ingredients in the saucepan over medium heat. Cook and stir until sugar is dissolved and carrots are glazed and tender. Serve immediately.

Serves 8

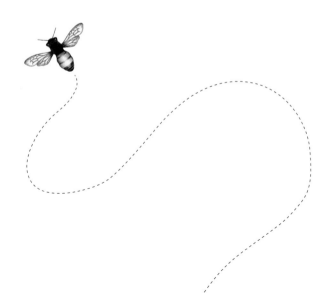

Glazed Ham and Fruit Tartlets

These beautiful little tartlets are an elegant main dish for a winter lunch.

DIRECTIONS

1. In medium bowl, combine cookie crumbs with butter and ⅓ cup honey; mix well. Divide among six 4-inch tartlet pans. Press onto bottom and ½ inch up sides; set aside.

2. In medium saucepan, heat olive oil over medium heat. Add onion; cook and stir for 4 minutes. Add pears; cook and stir for 3 minutes longer. Add ham and orange juice; cook and stir until liquid evaporates, about 5 minutes longer. Remove from heat.

3. Preheat oven to 350°F.

4. Stir orange marmalade into ham mixture; divide mixture among the tartlet shells. Top with cheese and drizzle each with half of the remaining honey.

5. Place shells on cookie sheet and bake for 25–35 minutes or until tartlets are glazed. Drizzle with the rest of the honey. Cool for 20 minutes, then serve.

Serves 6

INGREDIENTS

- 20 gingersnaps, crushed
- 2 tablespoons butter, melted
- ⅓ cup plus 2 tablespoons honey
- 1 tablespoon olive oil
- 1 onion, chopped
- 2 pears, peeled and diced
- 1 cup diced cooked ham
- 3 tablespoons orange juice
- ⅓ cup orange marmalade
- ½ cup shredded low-fat Swiss cheese

Honey Chili Chicken

INGREDIENTS

- 3 dried red chilies, roughly pounded
- ½ cup liquid honey
- Juice of 1 lemon
- 1 teaspoon soy sauce
- 2 teaspoons garlic paste
- 1½ pounds skinless, boneless chicken chunks
- Vegetable oil for basting

The contrasting tastes of the red chili and the honey make this Indian dish so delicious. The spiciness excites the taste buds, and the sweetness calms them and clears the mouth for the next bite.

DIRECTIONS

1. In a bowl, combine all the ingredients except the oil; mix well. Cover and refrigerate for at least 2 hours.

2. Preheat oven to 400°F.

3. Place the chicken on a baking sheet and roast for about 10 minutes.

4. Turn once and baste with oil. Roast for another 10 minutes or until cooked through. Serve hot.

Raspberry Vinaigrette

This pink vinaigrette dresses up a plain green salad, or try it drizzled over a mixed fruit salad for lunch. The honey thickens the mixture and softens the acidity of the raspberries.

DIRECTIONS

1. In food processor or blender, combine all ingredients. Process or blend until mixture is smooth.

2. Pour into small jar with tight lid. Cover and refrigerate up to 1 week, shaking the dressing vigorously before you use it.

1 cup, serves 8

- ¼ cup extra virgin olive oil
- ½ cup raspberry vinegar
- 1 cup frozen raspberries, thawed
- ¼ cup honey
- 2 tablespoons sugar
- ¼ teaspoon salt
- ⅛ teaspoon white pepper
- ½ teaspoon dried tarragon leaves
- ¼ cup raspberry jam
- 1 tablespoon Dijon mustard

HOMEMADE FLAVORED VINEGARS

It's easy to make flavored vinegars at home. Just select any fresh herbs, spices, or fruits and rinse and dry them well. Add them to good quality wine vinegars, cover tightly, and let stand for about a week before using. However, do not make homemade flavored oils; the risk of botulism is simply too great, even when they're refrigerated.

Honey Mustard Dressing

INGREDIENTS

- ½ cup chicken broth
- ½ cup salad oil
- 2 tablespoons Dijon mustard
- 1 tablespoon honey
- 2 tablespoons white wine vinegar
- 1 teaspoon minced onion
- Salt and pepper to taste

This smooth, spicy dressing is particularly good for salads with sliced chicken breast. It's healthy as well as delicious, because chicken broth takes the place of half the oil other recipes would use. Try using different oils to vary the flavor and weight of the dressing. Extra virgin olive oil is more flavorful than pure olive oil, which is lighter in taste.

DIRECTIONS

Combine ingredients in a blender until smooth. Adjust seasoning to taste with salt and pepper.

Serves 8

If you measure the oil called for in a recipe before you measure honey, molasses, or syrup the sticky ingredient will slide right out of the measuring cup. What if your recipe doesn't call for oil? Lightly oil the measuring cup before measuring the honey and you will have the same easy results.

Sweet

Honey can do wonderful and unexpected things with meats and vegetables. But its primary place has always been with dessert. And for good reason. The humble bee has created a substance as sweet as sugar, but far more complex, healthy, and versatile.

Here you'll find favorites from childhood, such as crisp homemade graham crackers and tender oatmeal cookies. You'll also find exotic recipes from faraway lands. Taste what the Italians do with honey in their addictive struffoli cookies, or their subtly sweet honeyed polenta. Take a culinary trip to Turkey with a treasured baklava recipe, or to Germany with their spicy Lebkuchen delicacy. You'll find sweet honey concoctions that you can drink, slice, or devour in one bite.

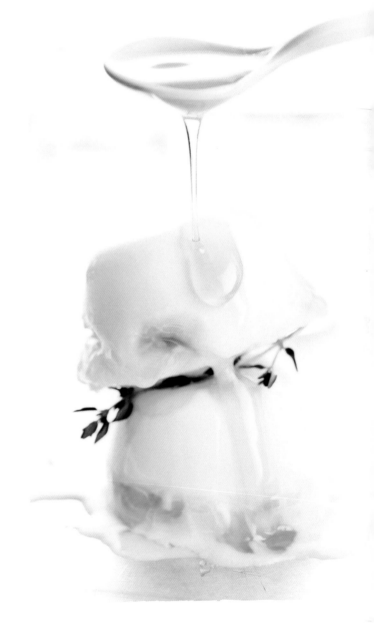

Sweet Honeyed Polenta

INGREDIENTS

- 5 cups water
- 1 cup milk
- 2 tablespoons unsalted butter
- 1¼ cups cornmeal
- ¾ cup honey

You may not be familiar with polenta, a ground cornmeal that's a staple of Italian cuisine, but it is the perfect showcase for an excellent batch of artisan honey. Polenta soaks up the flavor and moisture of the ingredients it's made with, and this porridge will take on the same rich taste as the honey you use. Depending on your personal tastes, this dish makes a filling breakfast or a unique dessert.

DIRECTIONS

1. Bring the water, milk, and butter to medium simmer in a large saucepan. Slowly whisk in the cornmeal, stirring constantly to avoid lumps. Reduce heat to low. Cook for 20–25 minutes, uncovered and stirring frequently, until thick and creamy.

2. Remove from heat, and stir in the honey. Serve hot.

Serves 10

Cinnamon Honey Butter

Honey butter should be a staple of any big meal. Spreading some on a hot fluffy roll, letting the butter melt into the warm bread before taking a bite—it's a divine experience that no one should miss. The cinnamon gives this spread a delightful kick that goes especially well with whole grains.

DIRECTIONS

1. In a small bowl, combine the softened butter with the honey.

2. Mix in the cinnamon until completely blended.

3. Store butter, covered, for up to 1 week (if there's any left!).

INGREDIENTS

- ¼ cup softened butter
- ⅓ cup honey
- ½ teaspoon cinnamon

Persimmon Split in Warm Honey Sauce

- 2 ripe persimmons, tops trimmed and split in half
- 2 scoops of your favorite ice cream
- ½ cup honey
- 1 tablespoon lemon juice
- 3 tablespoons crushed walnuts
- 1 cup whipped cream

If you haven't had a persimmon, seek it out. This fantastic fruit is available in the fall. They are ripe when quite soft. Although native to China, two varieties are available in the United States: a short, squat, round fruit and an elongated larger fruit. They are both suitable for this dish.

DIRECTIONS

1. Place the persimmons in a bowl and put the ice cream in the middle of the split fruit.

2. In a saucepan, combine the honey, lemon juice, and nuts. Heat until warm, and pour over the split.

3. Top with the whipped cream and enjoy.

Honeyed Figs on Warm Pita

This is a traditional breakfast in the Middle East, where people long ago discovered that the thick consistency of honey paired perfectly with the juicy pulp of figs.

DIRECTIONS

1. Place the yogurt in a colander lined with a coffee filter, and set over a bowl. Let drain overnight in the refrigerator. The next day, discard the water and place the yogurt cheese in a bowl.

2. Warm the pitas in a 350°F oven for 3 minutes. Spread with the yogurt cheese, drizzle with the honey, and top with the figs.

- 2 cups plain, whole yogurt
- 2 pita bread rounds
- 4 tablespoons honey
- 8 ripe figs, cut in half

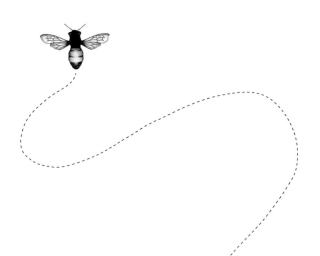

Easy Homemade Graham Crackers

- ¾ cup unbleached all-purpose flour
- 1½ cups whole wheat graham flour
- 1 teaspoon baking powder
- ½ teaspoon baking soda
- ½ teaspoon salt
- ¼ teaspoon ground cinnamon
- ¼ cup sugar
- ¼ cup brown sugar
- ½ cup cold unsalted butter, cut into pieces
- ¼ cup honey
- ¼ cup cold water
- 1 teaspoon vanilla or maple extract
- 1 tablespoon turbinado sugar

Your childhood memories are probably full of graham crackers—the crisp snap as you broke them across the perforated lines, the wholesome taste as you bit into a s'more. Honey adds a sweetness and a depth of flavor to what otherwise would be a bland bite.

DIRECTIONS

1. In a food processor, mix together dry ingredients and sugars (except turbinado sugar). Pulse until blended.

2. Add butter; pulse until mixture resembles coarse crumbs. Add honey, water, and extract; mix until dough forms a ball.

3. Roll dough ½ inch thick between two sheets of waxed paper. Chill 1 hour.

4. Preheat oven to 350°F.

5. Line a baking sheet with parchment paper. Roll chilled dough ⅛ inch thick; cut into desired shapes or squares. Prick holes in crackers with a fork; sprinkle turbinado sugar over tops.

6. Bake 15 minutes, or until lightly browned. Cool crackers completely.

Makes 48 crackers

Honey Oat Bran Bars

For this recipe, you can use plain bran flakes or raisin bran instead of the oat bran flakes. If using raisin bran flakes, just omit the raisins called for in the recipe, unless you like a lot of raisins.

DIRECTIONS

1. Grease 9" × 9" square pan; set aside.

2. Mix cereal, nuts, and raisins in a large bowl; set aside.

3. Bring butter, honey, and brown sugar to a boil over medium heat, stirring constantly.

4. Boil 5 minutes, continuing to stir constantly.

5. Pour over cereal mixture; stir to coat evenly. Spoon into prepared pan; press down gently. Cool 1 hour before cutting into bars.

Makes 16 bars

INGREDIENTS

- 4 cups oat bran flakes
- ½ cup chopped toasted pecans
- ½ cup raisins
- ⅓ cup unsalted butter
- ⅓ cup honey
- ⅓ cup firmly packed brown sugar

Struffoli

INGREDIENTS

- ¼ cup unsalted butter
- 2½–3 cups all-purpose flour
- ½ cup sugar
- ½ teaspoon salt
- 2 teaspoons baking powder
- 4 eggs, beaten
- 2 tablespoons lemon zest
- 1½ cups honey
- ¾ cup toasted almonds, chopped
- Candy sprinkles, optional

For this Italian holiday specialty, fried dough is dipped in boiling honey. The cookies are a lovely golden-brown hue, and just sticky enough to be easily stackable. Arrange a number of them into a pyramid for a festive occasion.

DIRECTIONS

1. Set electric fryer for 375°F. Melt butter; set aside.

2. Mix 2½ cups flour, sugar, salt, and baking powder in a large bowl. Make a well in center and add eggs, lemon zest, and melted butter.

3. Stir with a large spoon until dough leaves sides of bowl. Knead in rest of flour ½ cup at a time, until dough is no longer sticky.

4. Break off sections of dough; roll into pencil-sized logs. Cut into ¼-inch-long pieces; set aside. Roll pieces into balls and fry until golden.

5. Bring honey to a boil; boil gently 3 minutes. Add fried dough; stir until well coated. Remove balls from honey with a slotted spoon. Place on a platter; sprinkle with remaining ingredients. Form into a tall cone, wreath, or other shape while still warm. Cool completely.

Serves 8

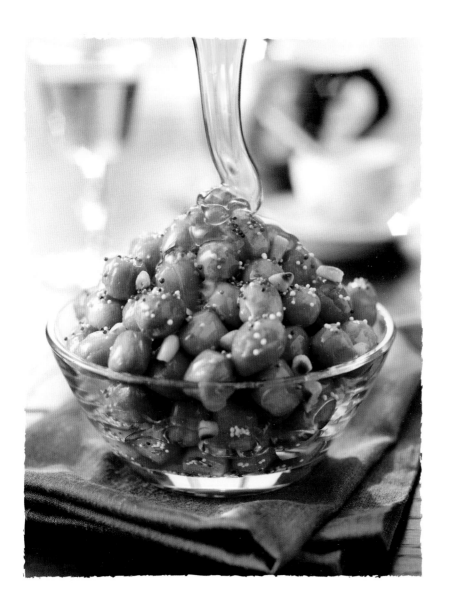

DEEP FRYING

When you are deep frying pastries and cookies, always start out with clean oil. A light type of oil with a high smoking point such as peanut oil is best. Allow the oil to reach the indicated temperature and then fry the dough a little at a time. When the dough begins to brown too quickly, it is time to change the oil.

Honey Balls

- ½ cup honey
- ½ cup peanut butter
- 1 cup confectioners' sugar
- 2 cups graham cracker crumbs

The graham cracker coating on these cookies elevates them from a simple dessert to a superb combination of consistencies. These cookies are no-bake, so they're an almost effortless cooking project for a lazy Sunday morning. Package them in small cellophane bags and tie with raffia for a sweet gift.

DIRECTIONS

1. Combine honey, peanut butter, and confectioners' sugar.

2. Roll into small balls.

3. Roll each ball in graham cracker crumbs.

4. Store at room temperature in an airtight container.

Makes 24 balls

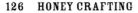

Honey Raisin Bars

These wholesome bars will satisfy your appetite on a woodsy hike or a summer camping trip. Cranberries can be substituted for the raisins if you like.

DIRECTIONS

1. Preheat oven to 375°F. Lightly grease 15" × 10" jelly roll pan.

2. Cream butter and sugars (except confectioners' sugar) until light and fluffy. Mix in eggs one at a time. Beat in honey and vanilla.

3. Whisk flours, baking powder, baking soda, salt, and spices together; gradually add to creamed mixture. Blend well; stir in remaining ingredients.

4. Spoon evenly in prepared pan; bake 18–20 minutes, or until done.

5. Cool. Cut into bars and roll in confectioners' sugar.

Makes 48 bars

INGREDIENTS

- ¾ cup unsalted butter
- ½ cup sugar
- ½ cup brown sugar
- 2 eggs
- ½ cup honey
- 1 teaspoon vanilla
- 1 cup all-purpose flour
- ½ cup whole wheat flour
- 1 teaspoon baking powder
- 1 teaspoon baking soda
- 1 teaspoon salt
- 2 teaspoons cinnamon
- ½ teaspoon freshly grated nutmeg
- ½ teaspoon allspice
- ¼ teaspoon cloves
- 1 cup raisins
- 1 cup walnuts, chopped
- Confectioners' sugar for rolling

Baklava

The moment this delicacy hits your tongue it will transport you to medieval Turkey, where the layers of phyllo dough and filling were a favorite dessert. Be sure to read the tips for using phyllo dough that are usually on the package. Thaw it in the refrigerator the day before you need to use it.

INGREDIENTS

- 1 pound chopped walnuts
- 1 teaspoon orange or lemon zest
- 1 teaspoon cinnamon
- 1 pound phyllo dough
- 1 cup butter, melted
- 1 cup white sugar
- 1 cup water
- 1 teaspoon vanilla
- ½ cup honey

DIRECTIONS

1. Preheat oven to 350°F. Butter 13" × 9" pan thoroughly.

2. Toss chopped nuts with zest and cinnamon; set aside.

3. Carefully unroll phyllo dough and cut stack in half so it fits in pan. Cover with a damp cloth.

4. Place two sheets of phyllo in pan; brush generously with butter. Repeat with two more sheets, until you have eight sheets layered in pan, brushing each layer with butter.

5. Sprinkle with 3 tablespoons of nut mixture. Top with two sheets of phyllo, brush with butter, then sprinkle with 3 more tablespoons of nuts. Continue building layers until nuts are used up. Top layer should consist of about eight layers of phyllo brushed with butter after every two layers.

6. With a sharp knife, cut almost all the way through baklava in four long rows, then diagonally to create diamond shapes. Do not cut through bottom layer until serving finished baklava. This will keep it from being soggy.

7. Bake 50 minutes.

8. Bring sugar and water to a boil, stirring until sugar is melted. Add vanilla and honey. Simmer mixture 20 minutes. When baklava comes out of the oven, immediately pour sauce over it. Let cool uncovered.

Makes 18 baklava "diamonds"

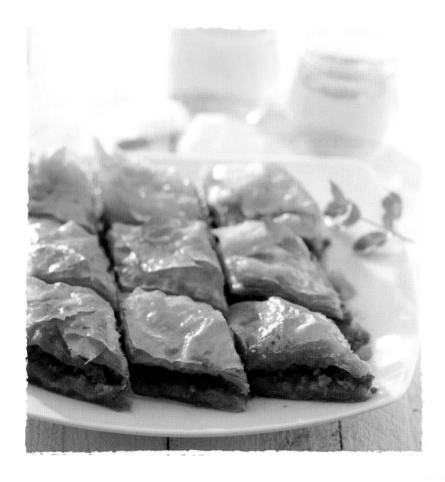

Lebkuchen

INGREDIENTS

- 1¼ cups sugar
- ¾ cup honey
- 2 tablespoons water
- 2 cups chocolate chips
- 1 cup almonds, chopped or slivered
- ½ cup candied citron or orange, chopped
- 2 eggs
- ¼ cup orange juice
- 2¾ cups all-purpose flour
- 2 teaspoons cinnamon
- 1 teaspoon cloves
- 2 teaspoons cardamom
- 1 teaspoon baking soda
- 1 teaspoon baking powder
- 3 tablespoons orange juice
- 1½ cups confectioners' sugar

These spicy German cookies need a few days to ripen after baking or the spices will taste too strong. The dough is very sticky to work with, but the finished product is worth it.

DIRECTIONS

1. Bring sugar, honey, and water to a rolling boil. Remove from heat; set aside to cool.

2. Stir honey mixture with chocolate chips, almonds, candied fruit, eggs, and orange juice.

3. Sift together flour, cinnamon, cloves, cardamom, baking soda, and baking powder; add to honey mixture. Cover bowl tightly; refrigerate 3 days.

4. Preheat oven to 325°F. Line 15" × 10" pan with parchment paper. Spread cookie dough evenly in pan.

5. Bake 35–40 minutes. Cool.

6. Mix orange juice and confectioners' sugar to make a thin frosting. Spread over tops of cookies. Store cookies in an airtight container.

Makes 48 cookies

Nut Butter and Honey on Whole Grain

Think beyond peanut butter and make your own spread for this delectable snack. The nut butter you'll make is less oily and far richer than what you would buy in a store.

DIRECTIONS

1. Purée the nuts until a smooth paste forms.

2. Spread onto bread and drizzle with honey.

Serves 6

- 2 cups nuts (shelled)
- 6 tablespoons honey
- 12 slices whole grain bread (toast if desired)

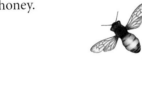

Date-Almond Tart

INGREDIENTS

- 1 cup flour
- 2 teaspoons olive oil
- 1 teaspoon ice water
- 1 cup chopped dried dates
- ½ cup chopped almonds
- ½ cup honey
- 1 cup plain nonfat yogurt
- ¼ cup confectioners' sugar

The honey in this recipe acts as a delicious bond for the tart's filling. For an added kick, use flavored yogurt with this recipe.

DIRECTIONS

1. Preheat oven to 375°F.

2. Mix together flour, olive oil, and ice water to form dough. Roll out dough into pie shell. Place in quiche or pie pan.

3. Mix together the dates, almonds, and honey. Place the date mixture in the center of the dough and loosely fold over pastry edges.

4. Bake for 20 minutes. Let cool and serve with yogurt and sprinkled confectioners' sugar.

Serves 6

Berry Fruit Dip

Serve this beautiful dip with seasonal fruit, baked unsalted tortilla chips, or plain sugar cookies.

DIRECTIONS

1. In food processor or blender, combine raspberries, strawberries, honey, orange juice, tofu, and salt; process or blend until smooth.

2. Place in small bowl; stir in dried cherries. Cover and chill until serving time, about 2–4 hours.

Serves 8

- 1 cup raspberries
- 2 cups chopped strawberries
- ¼ cup honey
- 2 tablespoons orange juice
- 1 cup silken tofu
- Pinch salt
- ½ cup chopped dried cherries

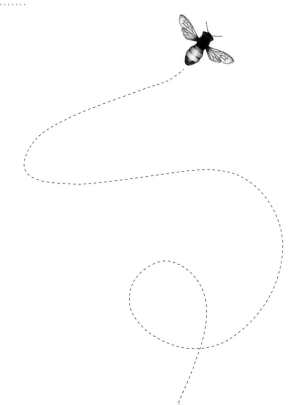

Honey Almond Cream Cheese Dip

- 8 ounces cream cheese, at room temperature
- 1 cup sour cream
- 2 tablespoons honey
- 1 teaspoon vanilla extract
- ¼ cup finely chopped toasted almonds
- 1 teaspoon Amaretto or almond liquor
- Finely chopped toasted almonds, for garnish

This is a delicious dip for fruits. Serve this accompanied by sliced apples, pears, strawberries, and grapes. If you need to cut the fruit more than a few hours before serving, dip apple and pear slices in a mixture of 2 tablespoons rice wine vinegar and 1 teaspoon honey. The acid in the vinegar will keep the apples and pears from browning, and the honey will take out the vinegar's tang.

DIRECTIONS

Combine all the ingredients (except the garnish) in a food processor fitted with a metal blade and process until well mixed. Transfer to a serving bowl and garnish with chopped almonds.

Serves 10

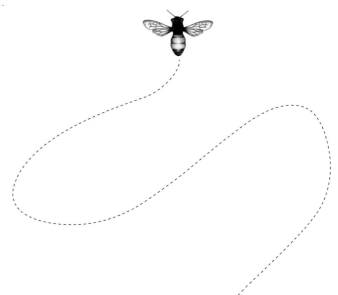

Oatmeal Peanut Butter and Honey Cookies

The sweet stickiness of honey and the smooth wholesomeness of peanuts make a popular combination.

DIRECTIONS

1. Preheat oven to 325°F.

2. In large bowl, combine butter and peanut butter; beat until smooth. Add brown sugar and beat well. Then stir in powdered sugar, honey, egg, egg whites, and vanilla.

3. Add the flours, baking powder, baking soda, and salt, and stir until a dough forms. Stir in oatmeal and oat bran, then add the dried fruit.

4. Drop dough by tablespoons onto a Silpat-lined cookie sheet. Bake for 12–16 minutes or until cookies are set. Cool for 5 minutes on cookie sheets, then remove to wire rack to cool.

Makes 48 cookies

INGREDIENTS

- ½ cup butter, softened
- 1½ cups peanut butter
- 1 cup brown sugar
- ½ cup powdered sugar
- ⅓ cup honey
- 1 egg
- 4 egg whites
- 2 teaspoons vanilla
- 1 cup all-purpose flour
- ⅓ cup whole wheat pastry flour
- ½ teaspoon baking powder
- ½ teaspoon baking soda
- ½ teaspoon salt
- 2½ cups regular oatmeal
- ½ cup oat bran
- 1 cup dried currants
- 1 cup dried cherries
- 1 cup dried cranberries

Pumpkin Puff Pie

INGREDIENTS

- 1 egg white
- ¼ cup sugar
- 1½ cups finely crushed graham crackers
- 2 teaspoons vanilla, divided
- 1 (¼-ounce) package unflavored gelatin
- 1 cup 1% milk, divided
- 2 egg yolks
- ½ cup honey
- ¼ cup brown sugar
- ¼ teaspoon salt
- 1½ teaspoons pumpkin pie spice
- 1 (15-ounce) can solid pack pumpkin
- 1½ cups nonfat frozen whipped topping, thawed
- ⅓ cup toffee bits

This dessert combines a light, airy pumpkin mousse with a crisp, crunchy pastry crust. The result is a splendid blend of texture that will delight all ages.

DIRECTIONS

1. Preheat oven to 375°F. Spray a 9-inch pie pan with nonstick baking spray that contains flour and set aside.

2. In medium bowl, beat egg white until soft peaks form. Gradually add sugar, beat until stiff peaks form. Fold in cracker crumbs and 1 teaspoon vanilla.

3. Spread into the pie plate, pressing onto bottom and up sides. Bake for 12–15 minutes or until set. Cool completely.

4. For filling, in small bowl, combine gelatin with ¼ cup milk. In large saucepan, combine remaining milk with egg yolks, honey, brown sugar, salt, and pumpkin pie spice. Heat until steaming. Stir in gelatin, and cook over low heat until gelatin and sugar dissolve.

5. Stir in the pumpkin and remaining 1 teaspoon vanilla and beat well until smooth. Let cool for 45 minutes. Fold the whipped topping into the pumpkin mixture and spoon into pie shell.

6. Cover and chill for 4–5 hours until firm. Sprinkle with toffee bits and serve.

Serves 8

Honey Swirled Pear Gelato

The floral notes of the honey and pear in this recipe dance together like bees buzzing around a flower.

DIRECTIONS

1. Combine milk, cream, sugar, ⅓ cup honey, and salt in a medium saucepan. Bring to boil. Remove from heat.

2. In a separate bowl, whisk egg yolks. Temper the yolks by adding half of the hot milk mixture into the eggs, whisking constantly. Add egg mixture to saucepan, and heat until thickened.

3. Add pear nectar, cardamom, and smashed pears.

4. Refrigerate at least 4 hours or overnight.

5. Add to ice cream maker and follow manufacturer's instructions for freezing. Stop the churning as soon as the gelato is just frozen. Swirl in the remaining ⅓ cup honey and freeze.

Makes 1 quart

INGREDIENTS

- 2 cups whole milk
- ½ cup heavy cream
- ⅓ cup sugar
- ⅔ cup honey, divided
- Pinch salt
- 4 large egg yolks
- 1½ cups pear nectar or purée
- ¼ teaspoon cardamom
- 1 (15-ounce) can pears, drained and roughly smashed

Lavender Honey Ice Cream

INGREDIENTS

- 1 cup whole milk
- 1¼ cups honey
- 3 tablespoons lavender buds (dried or fresh)
- ½ cup sugar
- Pinch salt
- 4 large egg yolks
- 2 cups heavy cream
- 2 teaspoons vanilla extract

Rich and creamy with floral notes, this ice cream soothes the senses and indulges the taste buds.

DIRECTIONS

1. In a small saucepan, combine the milk, honey, lavender buds, sugar, and salt. Stir over medium heat. Once simmering, remove from heat, cover, and allow to steep for 1 hour.

2. After 1 hour, strain milk mixture into a large measuring cup. Discard used buds and pour milk mixture back into pan. Reheat milk mixture over medium-low heat.

3. In a separate bowl, whisk egg yolks. Once milk mixture is hot, temper the yolks by adding half of the mixture into the eggs, whisking constantly. Add egg mixture to the saucepan, and heat until thickened.

4. Pour heavy cream into a large mixing bowl over an ice bath. Strain custard into the cream, stirring until cooled. Add vanilla extract; stir, and place in refrigerator until thoroughly chilled, about 5 hours or overnight.

5. Once chilled, add to ice cream maker and follow manufacturer's instructions for freezing.

Makes 1 quart

Mocha Chai Punch

The honey and cardamom in this recipe add a luscious twist to a traditional milk-tea punch. Use green or white tea for a lighter, but still delicious, festive drink.

DIRECTIONS

1. Pour the tea concentrate into large bowl or pitcher; set aside.

2. In large saucepan, combine sugar, honey, cardamom, cocoa powder, and milk and mix well with wire whisk.

3. Cook sugar mixture over medium heat, stirring frequently, until it just comes to a simmer. Pour into the tea concentrate and stir well.

4. Cover and chill for at least 24 hours.

5. When ready to serve, stir punch and pour into punch bowl. Add ginger ale and mix gently. Serve immediately.

INGREDIENTS

- 1 (16-ounce) bottle black tea concentrate
- ⅓ cup sugar
- ¼ cup honey
- ½ teaspoon ground cardamom
- ¼ cup cocoa powder
- 2 cups skim milk
- 1 (32-ounce) bottle ginger ale, chilled

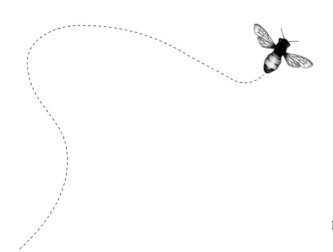

Homemade Honey Lemonade

- 5–6 large lemons
- 1¾ cups honey
- ½ gallon boiling water

This sweet, rich lemonade has little in common with the watered-down sugary version you would find in a supermarket.

DIRECTIONS

1. Scrub the lemons and halve them.

2. Squeeze the juice and pulp into a large bowl.

3. Add the honey, and pour half the water over it. Stir until the honey dissolves.

4. Add the lemon halves and the rest of the water.

5. Stir well, then cover and allow to cool.

6. Strain, squeezing out the juice from the lemon halves, and serve with ice.

Makes about 10 cups

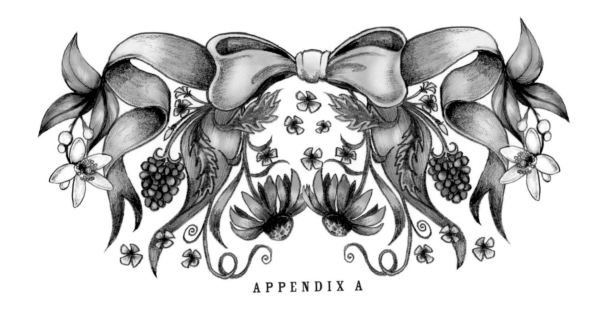

APPENDIX A

Resources

RESOURCE SITES

Botanical.com
A great resource for information on herbs.
www.botanical.com

Saponifier Magazine
Web magazine for the candle-making and soap-making communities.
www.saponifier.com

The Soap Dish Forum
An invaluable community of online soapmakers. (You must register to view the forum.)
www.soapdishforum.com

Beesource Beekeeping
Worldwide forum for beekeepers to share advice and experience.
www.beesource.com

Betterbee
Provides information on the state laws regarding beekeeping, as well as beekeeping clubs and associations across the country. Also a great supplier of beekeeping equipment.
www.betterbee.com

SUPPLIERS

Mann Lake Ltd.
Beekeeping supplier with a rewards program for frequent buyers.
www.mannlakeltd.com
1-800-880-7694

Dadant
A thorough and comprehensive catalog of tools and supplies for beekeeping and honey crafting —from wicks for candles to screens for hives.
www.dadant.com
1-888-922-1293

Walter T. Kelley Co.
Bees and beemaking supplies.
www.kelleybees.com
1-800-BEE-BUZZ

Honey Pacifica
Great resource for beeswax, an extensive array of honey, royal jelly, and propolis.
www.honeypacifica.com
1-562-938-9706

Bramble Berry
Large selection of supplies for crafting candles, soaps, and lotions.
www.brambleberry.com
1-360-734-8278

Milky Way
Catherine Failor's outstanding line of soap molds and stamps.
www.milkywaymolds.com
1-800-588-7930

Earth Guild
Basic molds, wicks, and wax for candle makers.
www.earthguild.com
1-800-327-8448

The CandleMaker
An excellent resource for wax and wicks.
www.thecandlemaker.com
1-888-251-4618

Camden-Grey
Essential oils and soap supplies.
www.camdengrey.com
1-305-500-9630

Natural Oils International
Excellent source of base oils and melt-and-pour soap bases.
www.naturaloils.com
1-805-433-0160

Wholesale Supplies Plus
Wide range of soap-making supplies, including airless pumps for liquid soap.
www.wholesalesuppliesplus.com
1-800-359-0944

The Scent Shack
Fragrance oils, essential oils, pigments, and more.
www.thescentshack.com
1-518-632-4802

Sweet Cakes
Extensive listings of soap-tested fragrance oils.
www.sweetcakes.com
1-952-945-9900

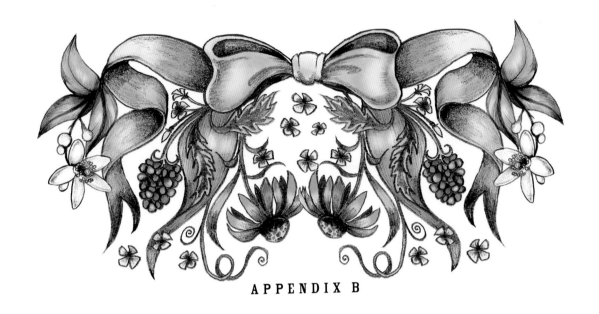

Tips on Beekeeping

If you haven't already ventured into the fascinating world of beekeeping, maybe the crafts in this book have convinced you that it's worthwhile. The decision to care for hives should not be taken lightly. Here is some basic information to get you started, but if you're interested in beekeeping, be sure to do thorough research before you begin.

Choosing the Right Hive Location

Honeybees can be kept almost anywhere that there are flowering plants that produce nectar and pollen. The best source of pollen and nectar should be within two square miles of your hive, the closer the better. Because bees actually use pollen and nectar to fuel their own energy, the farther they have to travel for it, the more they have to consume themselves. So, if you can place them closer to their food source, you can collect more honey.

Choose a site for beehives that is discrete, sheltered from winds, and partially shaded. Avoid low spots in a yard where cold, damp air accumulates in winter.

Position your hive so the entrance faces east. This way the early morning sun will alert the bees to the new day. The best position for a hive is where it will also have afternoon shade, shielding the hive from the summer sun. Shade, rather than sunlight, will give the bees more time to concentrate their effort on making honey, because they won't need to work at carrying water back and forth to cool the hive.

Basic Equipment

Here's what you'll need to build a hive and keep your own bees:

- **BOTTOM BOARD:** a wooden stand that the hive rests upon. Bottom boards can be set on bricks, concrete blocks, cinder blocks, or any stable base to keep the hive off the ground.
- **HIVE BODY OR BROOD SUPER:** a large wooden box that holds eight to ten frames of comb. In this space, the bees rear their brood and store honey for their own use. Up to three brood supers can be used for a brood nest.
- **FRAMES AND FOUNDATION:** frames hang inside each super or box on a specially cut ledge, called a rabbet. Frames keep the combs organized inside your hive and allow you to easily and safely inspect your bees. Frames hold thin sheets of beeswax foundation, which is embossed with the shapes of hexagonal cells. Foundations help bees to build straight combs.
- **QUEEN EXCLUDER:** a frame made with wire mesh placed between the brood super and the honey super, sized so workers can move between the brood super and the honey super, but keeps the queen in the brood super, so brooding will not occur in honey supers.
- **HONEY SUPERS:** shallow boxes with frames of comb hanging in it for bees to store surplus honey. The honey supers hold the honey that is harvested from the hive.

- **INNER COVER:** placed on top of the honey super to prevent bees from attaching comb to the outer cover. It also provides insulating dead air space.
- **OUTER COVER:** placed on top of the hive to provide weather protection.
- **SMOKER:** a beekeeper's best friend. A smoker calms bees and reduces stinging. Pine straw, sawdust, chipped wood mulch, grass, and burlap make good smoker fuel.
- **HIVE TOOL:** looks like a small crowbar. It is ideally shaped for prying apart supers and frames.
- **BEE SUIT OR JACKET, VEIL, GLOVES, AND GAUNTLET:** protective personal gear worn when working with bees. Generally you need light-colored overgear to keep your clothes clean and to create a barrier between you and the bees. Bees are not threatened by light colors, so the color of the suit makes a great difference as to whether the bees will attack or not. Thin, plastic-coated canvas gloves, rather than the stiff, heavy leather commercial gloves, are supple and allow you more movement. Gauntlets are long cuffs that slide over your gloves to keep bees from climbing up your sleeves.
- **ANKLE PROTECTION:** elastic straps with hook-and-loop attachments to prevent bees from crawling up your pants legs.
- **FEEDERS:** hold sugar syrup that is fed to bees in early spring and in fall.

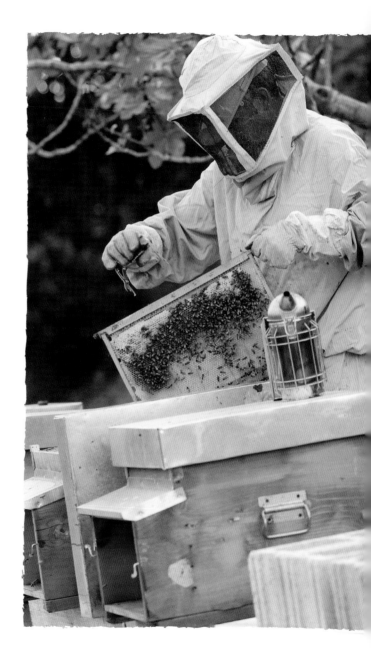

Obtaining Bees

Usually the best way to start keeping bees is to buy established colonies from a local beekeeper. Often a local beekeeper might even have a colony he or she wants to give away. It's better to get two colonies at the beginning, because that allows you to interchange frames of both brood and honey if one colony becomes weaker than the other and needs a boost. Have the beekeeper open the supers. The bees should be calm and numerous enough that they fill most of the spaces between combs.

Moving a hive is a two-person job. It's easiest to move a hive during the winter when it is lighter and populations are low. The first thing you want to do is close the hive entrance. You can accomplish this with a piece of folded window screen. Then look for any other cracks and seal them with duct tape. Make sure the supers are fastened together and the bottom board is stapled to the last super. Remember to open hive entrances after the hives are relocated. If you are buying the colonies, realize that the condition of the equipment usually reflects the care the bees have received. If you find the colonies housed in rotting hives, don't purchase them.

Your Hive, Year Round

You want your bees to be at their maximum strength before the nectar flow begins. This way, the created honey is stored for harvest rather than used to build up their strength. Feeding and medicating your bees should be done January through February. Because the queens will resume egg laying in January, some colonies will need supplemental feeding of sugar syrup. Note that not all beekeepers choose to feed their bees. It is considered good practice, if you do choose to supplement your hive's food supply, to do so only when necessary.

By mid-February, you should inspect your hives. You should be looking for population growth, the arrangement of the brood nest, and disease symptoms. If one of your colonies has less brood than average, you can strengthen it by transferring a frame of sealed brood from your other colony.

If you use two brood supers and find that most of the bees and brood are in the upper super, reverse the supers, placing the top one on the bottom. You want to do this because it relieves congestion. When a colony feels congested it swarms, looking for another place to live. If you only have one brood super, you will need to relieve congestion by providing additional honey supers above a queen excluder.

Annual requeening can be done in early spring or in the fall. Most keepers feel that requeening is one of the best investments a beekeeper can make. Young queens not only lay eggs more prolifically, but they also secrete higher levels of pheromones, which stimulate the worker bees to forage. In order to requeen a colony, you must find, kill, and discard the old queen. Then you need to allow the colony to remain queenless for 24 hours. After that period of time, you can introduce the new queen into her cage, allowing the workers to eat through the candy in order to release her.

By mid-April your colonies should be strong enough to collect surplus nectar. This is when you should add honey supers above the hive bodies. Add enough supers to accommodate both the incoming nectar and the large bee population. Adding supers stimulates foraging and limits late-season swarming.

During late summer and early autumn, the brood production and the honey production drop. At this point, you should crowd the bees by giving them only one or two honey supers. This forces bees to store honey in the brood nest to strengthen the hive.

Colonies are usually overwintered in two hive bodies or in one hive body and at least one honey super. Be sure that if you overwinter in one hive body and a honey super, you remove the queen excluder so the queen can move up into the honey super during winter. If your colony is light on stores, feed them heavy syrup (two parts sugar to one part water). Bees should have 50 to 60 pounds of stores going into winter. A hive with a full deep frame weighs 6 pounds and a full shallow frame weighs 3 pounds. You can pick up the frame to estimate the weight of the hive and stores. Never allow stores to drop below 12 to 18 pounds.

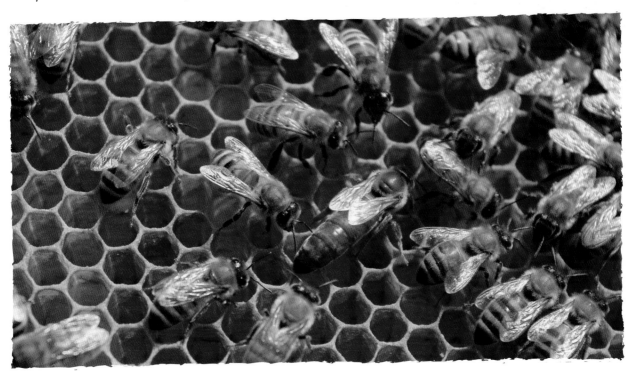

Common Problems

The common problems you encounter when raising bees are swarming, stings, and diseases and pests that can affect your hive.

SWARMING

You cannot always prevent bees from swarming. You can, however, make a swarm less likely by requeening your colony with a younger queen. You can also have a "bait hive" in place in case a swarm occurs. Bees will cluster within 100 feet of their old hive while the scout bees search for a new hive. A bait hive is simply an attractive home waiting for a swarm to discover.

STINGS

If you keep bees, you are going to get stung. You can reduce stinging greatly by taking precautions and wearing protective gear, using a smoker, and handling bees gently. However, the likelihood is that you're still going to get stung. If there is a chance you are allergic to bee stings, you do not want to keep bees. If you are not allergic, you probably will find, as most beekeepers do, that although stings still hurt, after a few stings there is generally less of a reaction.

HONEYBEE DISEASES AND PESTS

Honeybee broods and adults are attacked by bacteria, viruses, protozoans, fungi, and exotic parasitic mites. Additionally, bees and beekeeping equipment are attacked by a variety of insects. Some insects, like the wax moth, lay eggs on the equipment and their larvae gnaw boat-shaped indentations in the wooden frame or hive body to attach their silken cocoons. With heavy infestations, frame pieces may be weakened to the point of collapse. Some insects, like spiders, actually eat bees. Disease and pest control requires constant vigilance by the beekeeper. Contact local beekeepers to learn about the diseases and issues prevalent in your area and how to prevent and cure them.

Gathering Honey

It's best to harvest your honey on a sunny, windless day, because bees are calmest then. Remove the bees from the hive by blowing smoke into the hive opening. After a few minutes, pry the outer cover loose and lift it off. Blow more smoke through the hole in the inner cover. Now you can remove the inner cover. After the inner cover is removed, once again blow smoke into the hive to finally drive the bees downward and out of the way. Remove the super and pry the frames loose with the hive tool. Be careful not to crush any bees. A crushed bee releases a scent that stimulates other bees to attack. Gently brush off any bees that are clinging to the frames. A comb that is ready to be harvested should be about 80 percent sealed over.

Uncap the combs in a bee-proof location, such as a tightly screened room. Bees will want to take the honey, if they can get to it. Slice off the comb tops with a sharp knife warmed in hot water. A heavy kitchen knife is fine. It's best to use two knives, cutting with one while the other is heating. Once the honey is extracted, return the emptied combs to the hive for the bees to clean and use again. With care, combs can be recycled for 20 years or more.

Legal Requirements

All states have laws that pertain to keeping bees and registering hives. You need to understand the laws of your state before you begin beekeeping. For specific legal information, you can contact your county extension agent or your state department of agriculture.

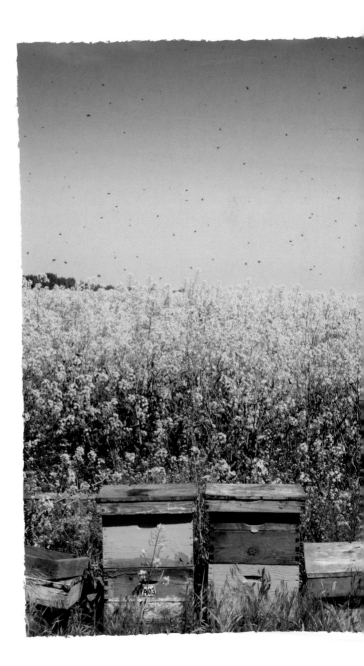

Index

Note: Page numbers in *italics* indicate projects. Page numbers in **bold** indicate food recipes.

Standard U.S./Metric Measurement Conversions

VOLUME CONVERSIONS

U.S. Volume Measure	Metric Equivalent
⅛ teaspoon	0.5 milliliter
¼ teaspoon	1 milliliter
½ teaspoon	2 milliliters
1 teaspoon	5 milliliters
½ tablespoon	7 milliliters
1 tablespoon (3 teaspoons)	15 milliliters
2 tablespoons (1 fluid ounce)	30 milliliters
¼ cup (4 tablespoons)	60 milliliters
⅓ cup	90 milliliters
½ cup (4 fluid ounces)	125 milliliters
⅔ cup	160 milliliters
¾ cup (6 fluid ounces)	180 milliliters
1 cup (16 tablespoons)	250 milliliters
1 pint (2 cups)	500 milliliters
1 quart (4 cups)	1 liter (about)
1 gallon	3.8 liters

WEIGHT CONVERSIONS

U.S. Weight Measure	Metric Equivalent
½ ounce	15 grams
1 ounce	30 grams
2 ounces	60 grams
3 ounces	85 grams
¼ pound (4 ounces)	115 grams
½ pound (8 ounces)	225 grams
¾ pound (12 ounces)	340 grams
1 pound (16 ounces)	454 grams

OVEN TEMPERATURE CONVERSIONS

Degrees Fahrenheit	Degrees Celsius
120 degrees F	49 degrees C
140 degrees F	60 degrees C
200 degrees F	95 degrees C
250 degrees F	120 degrees C
275 degrees F	135 degrees C
300 degrees F	150 degrees C
325 degrees F	160 degrees C
350 degrees F	180 degrees C
375 degrees F	190 degrees C
400 degrees F	205 degrees C
425 degrees F	220 degrees C
450 degrees F	230 degrees C

LENGTH

American	Metric
1 inch	2.54 cm
1 foot	30.48 cm

BAKING PAN SIZES

American	Metric
8 x 1½ inch round baking pan	20 x 4 cm cake tin
9 x 1½ inch round baking pan	23 x 3.5 cm cake tin
11 x 7 x 1½ inch baking pan	28 x 18 x 4 cm baking tin
13 x 9 x 2 inch baking pan	30 x 20 x 5 cm baking tin
2 quart rectangular baking dish	30 x 20 x 3 cm baking tin
15 x 10 x 2 inch baking pan	30 x 25 x 2 cm baking tin (Swiss roll tin)
9 inch pie plate	22 x 4 or 23 x 4 cm pie plate
7 or 8 inch springform pan	18 or 20 cm springform or loose bottom cake tin
9 x 5 x 3 inch loaf pan	23 x 13 x 7 cm or 2 lb narrow loaf or pate tin
1½ quart casserole	1.5 liter casserole
2 quart casserole	2 liter casserole

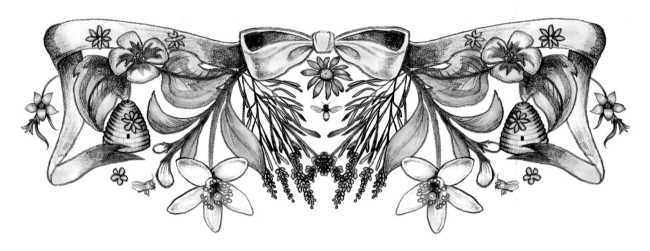

About the Authors

LEEANN COLEMAN operates Lee's Bees NJ, selling her honey and beeswax products to people all over the world. She is an all natural beepkeeper and organic gardener who owns Silver Spring Farm in New Jersey. Leeann is an officer in the Sussex County branch of the NJ Beekeepers Association. Learn more at *http://silverspringfarm.org*, and find her products at *www.leesbeesnj.etsy.com*.

JAYNE BARNES is a beekeeper, soap maker, and beeswax crafter who runs Honeyrun Farm near Williamsport, Ohio. Together with her husband Isaac they raise three children, keep 250 hives of bees, and produce seasonal raw honey, infused honey, cold-processed soap, and beeswax candles. Jayne is always inspired by the many versatile uses of honey and beeswax, and blogs about her experiences at *www.honeyrunfarm.blogspot.com*.